Luminos is the Open Access monograph publishing program from UC Press. Luminos provides a framework for preserving and reinvigorating monograph publishing for the future and increases the reach and visibility of important scholarly work. Titles published in the UC Press Luminos model are published with the same high standards for selection, peer review, production, and marketing as those in our traditional program. www.luminosoa.org

G

THE GEORGE GUND FOUNDATION
IMPRINT IN AFRICAN AMERICAN STUDIES

The George Gund Foundation has endowed
this imprint to advance understanding of
the history, culture, and current issues
of African Americans.

The publisher and the University of California Press Foundation gratefully acknowledge the generous support of the George Gund Foundation Imprint in African American Studies.

We Are Pregnant
with Freedom

REPRODUCTIVE JUSTICE:
A NEW VISION FOR THE
TWENTY-FIRST CENTURY

*Edited by Rickie Solinger (senior editor),
Khiara M. Bridges, Laura Briggs, Krystale E. Littlejohn,
Ruby Tapia, and Carly Thomsen*

1. *Reproductive Justice: An Introduction*, by Loretta J. Ross and Rickie Solinger
2. *How All Politics Became Reproductive Politics: From Welfare Reform to Foreclosure to Trump*, by Laura Briggs
3. *Distributing Condoms and Hope: The Racialized Politics of Youth Sexual Health*, by Chris A. Barcelos
4. *Just Get on the Pill: The Uneven Burden of Reproductive Politics*, by Krystale E. Littlejohn
5. *Reproduction Reconceived: Family Making and the Limits of Choice after Roe v. Wade*, by Sara Matthiesen
6. *Laboratory of Deficiency: Sterilization and Confinement in California, 1900–1950s*, by Natalie Lira
7. *Abortion Pills Go Global: Reproductive Freedom across Borders*, by Sydney Calkin
8. *Fighting Mad: Resisting the End of Roe v. Wade*, edited by Krystale E. Littlejohn and Rickie Solinger
9. *Fatal Denial: Racism and the Political Life of Black Infant Mortality*, by Annie Menzel
10. *The Pregnancy Police: Conceiving Crime, Arresting Personhood*, by Grace E. Howard
11. *Youth Organizing for Reproductive Justice: A Guide for Liberation*, by Chris A. Barcelos
12. *Queering Families: Reproductive Justice in Precarious Times*, by Tamara Lea Spira
13. *We Are Pregnant with Freedom: Black Feminist Storytelling for Reproductive Justice*, by Stacie Selmon McCormick
14. *From the Clinics to the Capitol: How Fighting Abortion Became Insurrectionary*, by Carol Mason

We Are Pregnant with Freedom

*Black Feminist Storytelling
for Reproductive Justice*

Stacie Selmon McCormick

UNIVERSITY OF CALIFORNIA PRESS

University of California Press
Oakland, California

© 2025 by Stacie McCormick

This work is licensed under a Creative Commons (CC BY-NC-ND) license. To view a copy of the license, visit http://creativecommons.org/licenses.

All other rights reserved.

Suggested citation: McCormick, S. S. *We Are Pregnant with Freedom: Black Feminist Storytelling for Reproductive Justice*. Oakland: University of California Press, 2025. DOI: https://doi.org/10.1525/luminos.236

Library of Congress Cataloging-in-Publication Data

Names: McCormick, Stacie Selmon, author.
Title: We are pregnant with freedom : black feminist storytelling for reproductive justice / Stacie Selmon McCormick.
Other titles: Reproductive justice ; 13.
Description: Oakland : University of California Press, [2025] | Series: Reproductive justice : a new vision for the 21st century; 13 | Includes bibliographical references and index.
Identifiers: LCCN 2024052555 (print) | LCCN 2024052556 (ebook) | ISBN 9780520422544 (cloth) | ISBN 9780520398795 (paperback) | ISBN 9780520398801 (ebook)
Subjects: LCSH: Afiya Center. | Reproductive rights—Texas. | Feminism—Texas. | Women, Black—Texas—Social conditions.
Classification: LCC HQ766.5.U6 M35 2025 (print) | LCC HQ766.5.U6 (ebook) | DDC 305.42089/96073—dc23/eng/20250203

LC record available at https://lccn.loc.gov/2024052555
LC ebook record available at https://lccn.loc.gov/2024052556

GPSR Authorized Representative: Easy Access System Europe, Mustamäe tee 50, 10621 Tallinn, Estonia, gpsr.requests@easproject.com

34 33 32 31 30 29 28 27 26 25
10 9 8 7 6 5 4 3 2 1

CONTENTS

Foreword

Reproductive Freedom Dreaming in Texas:
A Livable Black Futures Collective Statement

vii

Acknowledgments

xxvii

Introduction: Waterbreaking

1

1. Toward a Radical *We*: Decolonizing Sexual and Reproductive Health

31

2. Reproductive Justice: An American Grammar

58

3. Rememory: A Reproductive Justice Mixtape

71

4. Imagining Livable Black Futures
100

5. Abolition Medicine
120

6. Policing Black Birth
152

Epilogue: You Won't Break My Soul
175

Notes 189

Bibliography 215

Index 235

FOREWORD

REPRODUCTIVE FREEDOM DREAMING IN TEXAS

A Livable Black Futures Collective Statement

MARSHA JONES

STACIE MCCORMICK

D'ANDRA WILLIS

CERITA BURRELL

QIANA LEWIS-ARNOLD

HELEN ZIMBA

TAMBRA MORRISON

ALLISON TOMLINSON

And because we stopped telling stories we had this huge gap—Black folk been catching babies. Black folk been having abortions. Black folk been healing outside of a doctor's office. Black folk been doing this, but we stopped talking about it. So, to start telling stories again and to share stories, that's what's going to heal our nation. That's going to heal our people.

—Marsha Jones, founder and executive director of the Afiya Center

If Black women were free, it would mean that everyone else would have to be free since our freedom would necessitate the destruction of all the systems of oppression.

—*The Combahee River Collective Statement*

We are a collective of Texas-based reproductive justice activists, Black feminist health researchers, full-spectrum doulas, and HIV advocates who are holistically invested in the well-being of Black people. Though we've done this work well before 2021, our collectivity was established during the pivotal years of 2020 and 2021, which were rife with assaults on the bodily autonomy of womxn[1] and queer folk as well as the ongoing effects of Covid-19, which were disproportionately severe for Black folks. The state of Texas had just passed Senate Bill 8, the Heartbeat Bill,[2] which essentially banned abortion in the state, a move that would ultimately go national with the dismantling of *Roe v. Wade* as a result of the *Dobbs v. Jackson* decision. At the same time, Texas lawmakers were laying the foundation for Senate Bill 14, which criminalizes gender-affirming care (including hormone blockers and other supportive measures for transitioning queer youth). Black wombholders were giving birth in precarious situations, and we now know that the maternal mortality rates during this time were higher than average and that Black wombholders were most affected by these circumstances.[3] The heat from protests against socially sanctioned killings of Black folks, particularly Ahmaud Arbery, Breonna Taylor, and George Floyd, was still aflame in our communities. We were under attack, and stories became our weapon to fight back.

The Livable Black Futures Collective was formed primarily as a storytelling project designed to gather community stories as sources of knowledge for navigating our present circumstances and facilitating better futures. We looked to thinkers like Audre Lorde, who in her essay "Man Child" asserts that as a Black woman committed to a livable future, "I must examine all my possibilities of being within such a destructive system."[4] What possibilities for being existed for us when so much of our being was being attacked? Another key question we were concerned with was this: In naming our experiences of obstetric violence and institutional and medical racism, how could we imagine new possibilities of being and care that would enable Black futures? Through a fund provided by the American Council of Learned Societies and the Afiya Center in Dallas, Texas, which powers the Livable Black Futures Collective, we brought Black wombholders together (particularly those whose stories don't receive enough light, namely those who occupy marginalized identities and positionalities—economically and housing insecure, queer, nonbinary, formerly incarcerated, living with HIV, and more). We wanted to focus on these voices because we share an ethic to listen to those most affected and most marginalized. We had access to a great many accounts about issues like the Black birthing crisis from the perspective of Black, middle-class, cisgendered, and heteronormative women, but not enough from those who did not fit within those frames. And while we did not want to devalue the importance of those stories, we knew we had to bring all voices to the table to truly address the issues we face. In this respect, we speak in solidarity with Dorothy Roberts, who says, "Every indignity that comes from the denial of reproductive autonomy can be found in slave women's lives."[5] Roberts highlights that enslaved women were treated as exploitable commodities who experienced sexual and reproductive violence and holistic harm. We take our cue from Roberts's focus on those who are multiply marginalized as key to our conversations about freedom and bodily autonomy. We also take inspiration from the Combahee River Collective, which asserts: "If Black women were free, it would mean that everyone else would have to be free since our freedom would necessitate the destruction of all the systems of oppression."[6] Following their sentiment, we affirm that we cannot achieve full reproductive justice until the voices of the most marginalized Black wombholders are centered in our research and conversations.

The Afiya Center in Dallas, Texas, serves as a key space for us to develop our work because the organization supports Black folks who contend with the politics of disposability on many levels because of their social identities. Founded in 2008, the Afiya Center began as a vision of Marsha Jones and Mukamtagra Jendayi in response to an underserved and neglected population of Black womxn in North Texas. As HIV outreach workers, Jones and Jendayi identified a glaring gap in HIV messaging and the reception of such messaging by Black womxn. They knew they needed to offer a holistic approach to HIV prevention that addressed Black womxn's immediate challenges and circumstances; therefore, Jones and Jendayi created the Afiya Center to address a "lack of programs centered to assist Black womxn living in poverty and susceptible to the heightened prevalence of HIV/AIDS."[7]

Named after the Swahili word *Afiya*, which means physical, emotional, and spiritual health and wholeness, the Afiya Center is rooted in reproductive justice—the framework that takes a holistic approach to health and well-being, promoting the right to have a child, the right not to have a child, and the right to raise children in healthy and safe environments. The Afiya Center is guided by Audre Lorde's philosophy that "there is no such thing as a single-issue struggle because we do not live single-issue lives." Its logo represents the "morning star signifying a new day and the wheel of transformative forward movement."[8] Since its foundational beginnings with HIV advocacy and outreach work, the Afiya Center has grown tremendously and now addresses key areas of need for Black womxn and birthing people in Texas and beyond: maternal mortality and morbidity, HIV advocacy, abortion access, criminal justice reform, doula access, and more.

It also powers key initiatives: the Texas Black Womxn Reproductive Justice Summit, the Southern Roots Doula Collective, the Livable Black Futures Collective, and the Black Womxn's Advocacy Training Academy. To this day, it remains the only Black-led reproductive justice organization in North Texas and has been on the front lines of the fight for bodily autonomy in Texas. It was a key plaintiff in a 2021 case against Texas Senate Bill 8.[9]

NOTHING ABOUT US WITHOUT US

Rooted in key values of the Afiya Center, the Livable Black Futures Collective went about our work unapologetically centering marginalized Black voices in the issues facing us in 2021 and informed by prior struggles. The beauty of the Afiya Center is that the organization is composed of the people it serves, so being sure that the research was carried out in alignment with this principle was deeply important. We relied on researchers with experiential knowledge who could enact the care and connectivity that this project demanded. We knew that we could not approach our questions from a traditional academic stance. Additionally, we drew on Black feminist qualitative research strategies to develop our methodology.[10] Working as participant-researchers in the space, we engaged in a practice of sharing our investments and experiences with our participants as a form of relationality, as well as building trust and community among us. We also declared the space to be one that was shame- and stigma-free. Most critically, our budget philosophy for enacting this research was grounded in valuing the time and knowledges of our participants by paying them appropriately for their time and providing resources that would allow them to participate. We know that many barriers to inclusion in research studies are about potential difficulties of access to participation and about researchers' unwillingness or inability to provide support for participation. Our budget principle was that Black womxn/wombholders are worthy of investment and care, so, we paid a stipend for each session they participated in and provided childcare, food, and, if needed, transportation support. Sometimes the barriers to participation were so great, especially for those formerly incarcerated, that we had to use the Zoom platform. Even in those cases, we prioritized participants' safety, care, and privacy, supporting them remotely. Our key message to everyone in the space was and continues to be "You matter to us and we value you."

What follows are meditations from the founding members of the Livable Black Futures Collective—executive director Marsha Jones, Stacie McCormick, D'Andra Willis, Cerita Burrell, Qiana Lewis-Arnold, Helen Zimba, Tambra Morrison, and Allison Tomlinson. It is important to add that our collective has expanded, and this work has made possible the constitution of a Black feminist-led research team at the Afiya Center that also includes Amber Reid, TeQuan Penny, and Robyn Adams.

Below, each of us shares what motivates us to do our work and the power of storytelling for reproductive justice.

• • •

> What brought me here was I didn't see us. A good friend of mine told me, if you don't see what you're looking for, create it. I didn't see Black womxn being served and their stories being told, and I especially did not see that in Texas. So I created the Afiya Center.
> —Marsha Jones, executive director of the Afiya Center

I came to this work because I'm a Black womxn and if I was going to do the work of reproductive justice, I was going to do it from a Black womxn's perspective. After being in this work for so long, I noticed a lack of presence of Black womxn's voices. A key component to reproductive justice is telling our stories, our lived experience, and it felt like to me that Black womxn's stories were not being told by Black womxn.

This is especially true for HIV. It was the HIV component that brought us into this space. What brought me in was that a good friend of mine in the advocacy world told me, "If you don't see what you're looking for, create it." I didn't see Black womxn's stories being told, and I especially did not see that in Texas. Those stories need to be told regarding access to abortion and other forms of health care, including HIV services. Black womxn should be telling those stories free from stigma. And if those stories are going to be told, Black womxn should be telling them. Reproductive justice gave us the lens through which to tell our stories. For me, stories and data are interconnected. My goal has always been to bring the stories in conversation with the data. Mukamtagra Jendayi, who founded the Center with me, was very data driven, and her approach complemented mine in generative ways. I knew that once people told their stories, then the data would support those stories.

Livable Black Futures is an opportunity for people to tell their authentic lived story. It's not doctored. It's not fixed up. It is all of the womxn sitting at the table—those who are uber-articulate and those who don't always know what to say. The project has been especially validating of the work we do here at the Afiya Center. The Livable Black Futures Collective has created a space to collect the authentic lived experiences and stories of Black womxn, which is key to our work. That work has only just begun.

• • •

> We learn in community. We fight in community. We
> survive in community. We heal in community.
> We get free in community.
>
> —Stacie McCormick

As a scholar who was formally trained in the academy but was introduced to Black feminist thought through the Black women who poured into me during my childhood in Mississippi (on porches and in beauty salons, kitchens, churches, and schools), I had been searching for a way to practice my scholarship that would be authentic to me. Trained in Black literary study, I was intimately invested in exploring the power of language for Black folks, especially as it was represented in Black feminist writing. I knew that the work I wanted to do did not exist in the academy alone—I needed to be in community. I wanted that work to benefit more than just me. When I found myself dealing with a loss of twin boys while I was writing my dissertation on Black womxn's literary representations of bodily pain, I felt this need for community even more deeply. Once I began my career as an academic, my research focus moved from the visual, literary, and performance resonances of slavery's afterlives to the continuing resonances of those afterlives for Black people and just what can be done about it. Reproductive justice was and remains the answer. For me, storytelling became a way to bridge the work I was doing in literary study and put it in conversation with the stories being told in the everyday—stories that weren't formally documented but needed to be heard. The Afiya Center welcomed me into the space as a partner in this work. I am deeply grateful for this and have grown so much as a scholar as a result.

    I see shared storytelling as key to building community and advancing freedom. We learn in community. We fight in community. We survive in community. We heal in community. We get free in community. The work we've done in the Livable Black Futures Collective, which draws on the critical power of storytelling espoused by reproductive justice trailblazers such as Loretta Ross, Marsha Jones, and Byllye Avery, has already affirmed this for me, and this book is a testament to its possibilities. Black feminist writers like Assata Shakur, Toni Morrison, bell hooks, Audre Lorde, and others use language as a conduit for freedom. As a humanities scholar, I want to see what is possible when we close the loop, studying and taking inspiration from Black feminist theory, memoir, poetry, and various forms of narratives as a key to articulating our own. I'm also inspired by Byllye Avery, who says, "When women make their stories public, without the shame and embarrassment that keep us silent about our health, we become active participants in our health, and those who listen to them and support them benefit as well."[11] I have seen firsthand the truth of this and the critical need to continue giving womxn/wombholders a platform to share their stories.

• • •

> It is critical that we share other possibilities. When we tell our stories, it changes policy. It creates programs for us to get the health care we need, and it promotes care for the next generation.
> —D'Andra Willis

My personal birthing journey and increasing awareness of Black maternal mortality and morbidity led me to do birth justice work at the Afiya Center. I remember vividly being at a meeting led by the Afiya Center. I was pregnant at the time and had just had a baby, and I just cried because I kept thinking I wouldn't make it to raise my child or birth the one I was due to have, so from there I went on a quest to make it so Black womxn wouldn't feel that despair.

I now have three children, and I have become a full-spectrum doula. I now work for the Afiya Center as our birth justice program coordinator and HIV advocate.

I wanted to do more research into Black womxn's stories because I knew our voices were not being heard. Whether because of structural racism or our own silence from not being encouraged to tell our stories, they just weren't being raised up. I think specifically about Black womxn and fibroids. I thought it was just common and accepted. I thought that at forty you would get a hysterectomy because so many womxn in my family and community experienced that. It is critical that we share other possibilities. When we tell our stories, it changes policy. It creates programs for us to get the health care we need, and it promotes care for the next generation.

When we share our stories, we learn about womb health, food rituals we pass down within our family, and more. We learn how to build self-advocacy. It allows us to advocate for our rights and our health. It is important to not just hear the stories of Black womxn but to trust and believe them. We can use these stories to produce data, publications, and further research so that those coming after us don't have to experience what we experienced. That is my hope for my own girls, ages five and three, to be able to have a playbook and have a different experience.

・　・　・

> As I continue to grow in this work, I see the necessity of telling our own stories as Black womxn and leveraging our voices to shape our own narratives about our lives—not allowing other folks to tell those stories. This is legacy work.
> —Cerita Burrell

I'm in this work because of the Afiya Center. I grew up in Southern California, and I didn't grow up around many Black folks, but I knew that my environment was inherently incorrect. I could not understand why I was in spaces, particularly in school, where no one else looked like me. It made me aware of social inequities and created within me a yearning to be around my people and be in connection with them. I knew the system around me was not for me, but I still felt under the pressure of living the "American Dream" that in order to get ahead you have to have all these things. I got my degree that I don't fully use because I thought that was the only way to get ahead, so it took me a while to pursue the things that mattered to me. I eventually moved to Texas, and I was introduced to Marsha Jones and the Afiya Center through a community project I was working on. I also had heard about AIDS and HIV, but I realized I didn't know as much as I would like to know. I was fascinated by how Marsha talked about Black womxn and how they were affected because really the conversation was mostly about gay men, so she brought a kind of intersectionality to it.

Another piece that fascinated me was that the Afiya Center was bringing economics and HIV into the conversation. So that was another thing that made me want to be a part of this. It gave me the opportunity to expand my knowledge and even understand the work of nonprofits, which was the work I wanted to get into. I feel like the beauty of the Afiya Center is that you get opportunities without having to be blocked because you don't have certain requirements or formal training. You are able to do the things you know you are capable of doing, so I was able to come into the world of reproductive justice and do the work while I was also learning things. I also had to learn how to deconstruct and shed white supremacy—seeing possibilities for work culture (understanding that two things can exist at the same time and that it doesn't have to be an either/or but can be a both/and) that are not the standard ideas. I continue to learn and grow: for instance, I am growing my knowledge around storytelling and the necessity of telling our own stories as Black womxn and leveraging our voices to shape our own narratives about our lives rather than allowing other folks to tell those stories.

Seeing the journey of Livable Black Futures has been beautiful and has even made me think about my own story. Sometimes I'll think to myself, oh my story is not as interesting, but that's not true because "your story is your story and so that's your truth." This is legacy work.

• • •

> This journey is a way of me honoring my ancestors. I always understood the work of storytelling as an act of defiance and cultural preservation because it's a key part of Black culture—our oral traditions. I have seen the power of this work firsthand.
> —Qiana Lewis-Arnold

Coming into the Afiya Center and birth justice work was an overall life calling. I've always kind of flowed somewhere in the space of activism, social justice, and birth work. That's how I landed at the Afiya Center, doing the work. As I've worked in this space more, I have seen how critical storytelling is for our people. For me, when you think about the enslaved, we understand that our ancestors couldn't write down their experiences because it wasn't safe. Some of them couldn't read. Some of them couldn't write, and a lot of them could read and write but couldn't reveal that. They also had their ancestral languages, but much of their journey wasn't written down.

They have been trying to erase these realities out of the history books, so much of the Livable Black Futures work was a way for me to honor my ancestors. I always understood the work of storytelling as an act of defiance and cultural preservation because it's a key part of Black culture—our oral traditions. I have seen the power of this work firsthand. It was like a spark that lit a flame in all of our participants. This project was so empowering for our participants. Just about everyone who participated has gone on to do their own projects centered on the health and healing of Black folks. It's amazing to just watch it work in real time. The impact that this work has had cannot be overstated. It gave words to the desires of Black womxn and black people, black wombholders in our community. Our Bill of Rights was transformative. We shared the tools in community, and they took those tools and did the work. It's so important that we tell our stories and create spaces where stories are told because that's where the healing happens, and that's how the work continues. Through our collective, the "Black Wombholders' Bill of Rights," and the critical space that we provided, we organically made it possible for people to come together and have a conversation and work through their trauma. We gave them a language and tools, and they took that and moved it forward.

• • •

> My anger at injustices to Black womxn with HIV motivated me to look for a better way and a way to make space for others that I didn't see out there.
> —Helen Zimba

What brought me into this work and the Afiya Center and really HIV work as a whole was that I was angry. I was angry with how things were being done and what I was being told. In the days when I began my HIV work, there was a lot of misinformation. I was reading books that would tell me what would happen to you, and it wasn't making sense. I wanted to know more, so my anger motivated me to look for a better way and a way to make space for others that I didn't see out there.

I felt like Black womxn were not being served, so I saw the Afiya Center as a space that was doing that. I happened to meet Marsha in the '90s when I was still figuring out where I wanted to be in this work, and I knew the Afiya Center would be a space for me to do the kind of work I felt was needed.

That also connects to the importance of telling our stories. For example, for a long time I didn't think I was a birth worker, but I realized I have been doing birth work for a while. I just didn't have a title for it. It was when I witnessed the work of a doula who was helping my daughter when she was having a baby, and I realized I was doing the same thing for her and others. That's why telling our stories is so important: because I didn't even know this was the work I was doing until I connected with others who helped me see that. Our stories need to be told by us. In the Livable Black Futures Collective we have been taking our stories and putting them into life. Every time someone shares something, it is often something others can relate to, even across generations. Some of us in the group had children a long time ago, but it was helpful to share our stories with others. And unfortunately some of the things that happened to us then are still happening now, so we need to share to help people navigate their current circumstances. In our work in the Collective, the process of people exchanging stories, hearing each other, and being supportive to each other is so important to me. There's a lot of empowerment going on, a lot of support, and to me it has become like a sisterhood.

• • •

> We have to tell the stories passed down to us by our grandmothers, grandfathers, mothers, and so on. This is community work. It is how we come together. It's how we heal. It's how we learn. It's how we grow.
>
> —Tambra Morrison

Working here at the Afiya Center is in many ways like a full-circle moment. I went to a womxn's event at David's Chapel Church where I saw Ms. Marsha talking about what she does here and letting people know how to volunteer. So I signed up for what I thought would be a volunteer role, and I was opened up to so much more. I was learning about abortion care, slavery, and period health from an ancestral perspective. I also joined as a participant in Livable Black Futures, and that was also a full-circle moment. I saw a vision for a career outside of my workplace at the time. I was making pretty decent money, and Ms. Marsha connected with me about working at the Afiya Center. Initially I was nervous, but I prayed and I felt God say, "Do it." I've been here, and it's been really powerful. When I joined, I realized I was actually in the right place and I knew more about reproductive justice than I'd thought. I feel that it was a divine reason for me being here.

My time participating in the Livable Black Futures storytelling work showed me that we can't sit on our hands, especially not this current generation. It's a life-or-death situation out here. We have to tell the stories passed down to us by our grandmothers, grandfathers, mothers, and so on. This is community work. It is how we come together. It's how we heal. It's how we learn. It's how we grow. We need to keep our ancestors' stories alive because they are still relevant. By telling our stories, we don't see ourselves as simply individuals. We see ourselves in connection. A lot of people have been or are going through what you've been through, and not only that, there are people out here fighting for you, people who have been on the front lines to get justice and change that we need.

• • •

> Through our work, we affirmed that storytelling has the power to heal in the reproductive justice community and that healing can come from within rather than from outside the community.
> —Allison Tomlinson

I wouldn't have initially considered my work advocating for, researching on, and working with incarcerated mothers birth justice work. However, I have come to understand that companioning womxn/mothers along the maternal and reproductive journey, even through incarceration, is a part of birth justice work. Often these womxn are the most forgotten and medically neglected. I came to this work through exposure to the truly abhorrent conditions that many incarcerated, especially Black and Latinx, womxn endure during incarceration, whether pregnant, birthing, or experiencing gynecological and obstetric issues.

As a mental health professional, I feel that it is important to raise up the impact of storytelling on mental health. I believe that storytelling, as it has been theorized, has a special place in the Black experience. We pass down many traditions and values through oral communication. We have also maintained that telling our story is healing and restorative for our community. There are schools of thought that use "narrative therapy," which is simply storytelling and reauthoring your story in a way that empowers. I believe that we learned storytelling has the power to heal in the reproductive justice community. Healing can come from within rather than from outside the community.

The Livable Black Futures Collective has created awareness about the need for a space for Black womxn to heal and be liberated within the community. I think this project has taught womxn in the service community that simply telling their story and not holding in the pain can be meaningful and helpful for themselves and others. Often we suffer in silence because no one has invited us to share our hurts and pain. I believe this project gave womxn a space and community to work on healing through shared experience. It reduced the stigma and shame of what they had experienced because they learned it wasn't just them who had been treated with ill regard and violence. Commiseration in the shared experience of inequity made it less personal. It externalized the problem and put it back in the correct context.

This project expanded knowledge on what is inclusively reproductive justice work (especially from a research perspective). There is much work to do to replicate it and make its results as well as these kinds of spaces more accessible for communities across the country.

. . .

OUR FREEDOM DREAMS

One of the key components of our storytelling work is to harness the power of the Black radical imagination. We work to envision what people think is impossible and move it toward reality. That is why, even amid all the oppressive contexts we face in the state of Texas, we believe we can create the world we want to see. In his work *Freedom Dreams and the Black Radical Imagination,* Robin D.G. Kelley asks, "What are today's young activists dreaming about?"[12] He also asks, "What are they fighting for?" Kelley affirms that freedom and love are the most powerful and revolutionary ideas available to us, but deep engagement with them on a sociopolitical level remains necessary. This speaks to our work in many ways because it is through storytelling, both in the imaginative work of others and in our own stories and the stories of those within the community, that we dream about the world we want and how we must fight for it. We dream of a world for Black womxn and birthing people that is safe, supportive, communal, well-resourced, and free. We want Black women and birthing people to feel safe no matter how they choose to give birth. We want them to experience a system that cares for them at all stages of the reproductive journey and respects the decisions they make for their own bodies and children. We want them to experience the joy of birth in community free from stigma. We especially want this for those living with HIV. We want those incarcerated to be able to get the support they need. We want them to be fully resourced, safe, and happy. Most importantly, we want them to be able to be unapologetically themselves in whatever setting they are in, pregnant or not. We invited our storytellers of the Livable Black Futures Storytelling Project to cocreate what we call a "Black Wombholders' Bill of Rights." It is an expression of our collective desires and freedom dreams for Black reproductive and sexual health. This document is a guide, a manifesto, and an evolving statement about what Black womxn and birthing people need to achieve care that is safe, supportive, communal, well-resourced, and free. We end with this as a foundation for the conversations that unfold in this book. *Asé.*

BLACK WOMBHOLDERS' BILL OF RIGHTS

- I have the right to choose *not* to have children at any point in my life.
- I have the unlimited right to an abortion at any gestational point in the pregnancy.
- I have the right to a judgment-free experience with health care providers and judgment-free conversations about sexual and reproductive health in my community.
- I have the right to a safe and compassionate gynecological health care experience.
- I have the right to receive information about *all* of the options available to me as they relate to my sexual and reproductive health.
- I have the right to make the best choice for me at *any* age!
- I have the right to care that is not informed by ableism or race-based medicine.
- I have the right to gynecological care that is not influenced by homophobia, transphobia, or any other normative perspective that does not consider my identity.
- I have the right to be called by my chosen name and not my given name during medical appointments.
- I have the right for my son to receive a thorough education on his sexual and reproductive health and rights.
- I have the right to supportive, shame-free, and antisexist community conversations about my sexual and reproductive health.
- I have the right for my voice to be heard free from retaliation.

ACKNOWLEDGMENTS

I owe a great deal to many people for the production of this book. When I began researching storytelling and reproductive justice, I knew this work was important to me and needed to be in the world. However, I did not anticipate how much this book would mean to so many with whom I am fortunate to be in community. Since I've taken up this work, much has transpired politically, particularly the overturning of *Roe v. Wade* and the ongoing tumult in its aftermath, especially in states like Texas, where I reside, and in states that have all but banned abortion. Being able to connect with all those who have provided support and community as I wrote this book has been invaluable to me.

I thank my children, Zoe and Jackson, as well as my twin boys, Leroy and Sylvester (named after their great-grandfathers), who were born too early to live outside of my womb but who left an indelible mark on my heart. I also thank my husband, Demetrius, for walking with me along this journey and encouraging me to turn my grief into power. I am so thankful to be doing life with you. My mother, Jana Selmon, and my mother-in-law, Earlean

McCormick, remain so valuable in the support of this work. My sister, Angela Sinclair, has been everything to me, providing me with loving accountability and encouragement when I needed it. I thank my father, Ezell Riley, my bonus mom, Gladys Riley, and my brothers, Sidney and Isaiah, for offering their support as well. I dedicate this work to my grandmothers, Lillie Pearl Selmon and L. G. Riley, whom I lost in 2018 and 2020, respectively. Their legacy continues to be my North Star.

I am immensely grateful to the University of California Press's Reproductive Justice Series editors, Khiara Bridges and Rickie Solinger, who believed in this project and helped me to bring it into being. Not only did they serve as key voices in the early stage of this work, but their scholarship also provided inspiration for the kind of work I want to do in the world. They, along with Naomi Schneider and Aline Dolinh, as well as the staff at University of California Press, have been patient, efficient, and deeply supportive.

The staff at the Afiya Center in Dallas, Texas, anchored this work. This book would not have been possible without them. I often say that their work as doulas applied to this book because they supported me in bringing it to life. Executive director Marsha Jones, D'Andra Willis, Qiana Arnold, Helen Zimba, Allison Tomlinson, and Cerita Burrell served as the first iteration of the Livable Black Futures Collective. We have grown since then and have welcomed Amber Reid, TeQuan Penny, Tambra Morrison, and Robyn Adams into this work. I am so excited about what we will continue to do together. Thank you for showing me what is possible when you do your work unapologetically and authentically.

I am fortunate to have fellow scholar-friends who have been with me on the journey: Rhaisa Williams, Aneeka Henderson, Nessette Falu, Tonya Foster, Jallicia Jolly, Samantha Henry, Kyrah

Brown, Meryleen Mena, Felecia Bevel, Michelle May Curry, and Therí Pickens. You all are brilliant and amazing people, whom I learn from all the time. My Texas Christian University colleagues are also dear to me, and I thank them for their community and support: Layne Craig, Bonnie Lucero, Lisa Smant, Brandon Manning, Grace Vargas, Shari Mackinson, Jasmine Jackson, Sam Davis, Theresa Gaul, and the RECC Writing Squad. I can't say enough about how grateful I am to have you all as colleagues.

My students have also been elemental in the development of my work. I give deep gratitude to Victoria Washington and Jacora Johnson, who served as research assistants for this book. Angela Mack (once a student and now a PhD graduate) and Kelly Franklin, I appreciate your keen interest and your being conversation partners with me. Also, the students in my Spring 2023 undergraduate Reproductive Justice course and my fall 2022 graduate Contemporary African American Literature course were thoughtful and engaged voices as I shared my work and studied alongside them.

The American Council of Learned Societies was key in the development of this project. Their financial support through the Mellon/ACLS Scholars and Society Fellowship provided me with resources and community—helping me enact the vision I had for this work. Desiree Barron-Callaci and John Paul Christy along with the ACLS staff were encouraging and offered great guidance for how my scholarship could be enacted in the world. My fellow recipients of the Mellon/ACLS Scholars and Society Fellowship, namely Treva Lindsey and Rachel Bloom-Pojar, remain inspirational for me as I continue. I also thank TCU and Dean Sonja Watson for providing research funding support via the Mid-Career Faculty Summer Research Grant in the Addran College of Liberal Arts.

Thank you to each and all for being fellow travelers (and often guides) on this path.

INTRODUCTION

Waterbreaking

> You know, they straightened out the Mississippi River in places, to make room for houses and livable acreage. Occasionally the river floods these places. "Floods" is the word they use, but in fact it is not flooding; it is remembering. Remembering where it used to be. All water has a perfect memory and is forever trying to get back to where it was. Writers are like that: remembering where we were, what valley we ran through, what the banks were like, the light that was there and the route back to our original place. It is emotional memory—what the nerves and the skin remember as well as how it appeared. And a rush of imagination is our "flooding."
>
> —Toni Morrison, "The Site of Memory"

> Movements for social justice are rivers.
>
> —Eesha Pandit

Black storytelling carries the force of water. It flows with memory. It can force a reckoning. It can move one to tears. It can engender life through its presentation of possible worlds imagined by a deeply oppressed people who refuse their oppression. This book is about my journey as a researcher, community advocate, and

Black birthing person to explore how the work of Black storytelling serves as a form of resistance to present-day and historical attacks on bodily autonomy, something deeply felt for Black people, whose lives have been subject to death-dealing, anti-Black social structures and surveillance of the state. I was especially keen to learn how Black birthing people were using storytelling to navigate the political landscape of 2020, where the ground shifted on so many issues. Covid-19 had laid bare for the world racial health inequities, and the racial reckonings in the aftermath of the death of individuals such as George Floyd and Breonna Taylor animated the American public around police violence in ways previously unseen. Alongside these issues, lawmakers in places like Texas (where I currently live) and Mississippi (my ancestral home) were laying the groundwork to challenge *Roe v. Wade*, resulting in the 2022 *Dobbs v. Jackson* decision[1] that would ultimately overturn what was once considered settled law. Additionally, gender-affirming care for queer and trans folk continues to be under attack, and organizations like Moms for Liberty have set their sights on education and stories as a part of the effort to turn back the clock on any type of racial or gender progress.[2] I write this reflection in the aftermath of the Supreme Court effectively ending affirmative action[3] and the Texas legislature prohibiting the funding of diversity, equity, and inclusion initiatives at public colleges and universities.[4] It is a dangerous onslaught.

Black birthing people sit squarely in the precarious intersections of this litany of social and political harms. Not only are they contending with alarmingly high rates of Black maternal mortality, but they also face difficulty parenting in environments where Black children are affirmed, safe, and healthy because these are becoming so elusive. When taken together, the above developments constitute a wholesale attack on reproductive justice, which is "the human right to maintain personal bodily autonomy, have children, not have children, and parent the children we have in safe and sustainable communities."[5] When we consider how every aspect of the tenets of reproductive justice is being actively undermined, there is a need to take an all-of-the-above approach to combating these efforts. As I saw the mobilization of communities via protests, political action, and other forms of advocacy, I was curious about the role that storytelling plays in this fight. Loretta Ross asserts that "storytelling is a crucial part of reproductive justice theory, an act of reclamation and resistance."[6] For Ross, storytelling is an act of subversion and resistance that militates against the onslaught of anxiety and the internalizing of oppressive ideas within ourselves due to harmful encounters with the medical-industrial complex.[7] Because I am a literary scholar who researches various dimensions of Black expressive culture, Ross's words resonate with me deeply. Black people have used storywork historically as a way to fight against oppression. Whether in slave narratives, sermons, performance and visual art, or speculative fiction, the Black radical imagination[8] has been key to liberation. This book is an attempt to document the contemporary manifestations of these practices and their advancement of reproductive justice and liberation. *We Are Pregnant with Freedom: Black Feminist Storytelling for Reproductive Justice* contends that Black feminist storytelling serves as a key site for advancing and expanding the underlying tenets of reproductive justice. This book points to the storytelling work of Black writers, activists, advocates, artists, and community members as a form of critical knowledge making, resistance, and imagining of new paths for healing and care. Black women and birthing people are often the most marginalized and most affected by gynecological and obstetric harm, yet their voices are often overlooked in broader medical discourse. Through my exploration of Black feminist storytelling for reproductive justice, I throw light on an archive of both injury and survival, a counter to the institutional medical record, and a vision for the future rooted in freedom.

THE PERSONAL AND THE POLITICAL

More than just academic, this work is personal for me because I am on my own healing journey from medical trauma and harm. While I was a graduate student, I became pregnant with twins. After the shock and joy of seeing two bean-shaped fetuses moving around on the ultrasound, I began to settle into the idea of being an academic and mother of what I would learn were twin boys. My husband and I began picking names and planning our future as parents. However, at twenty weeks, I learned that my cervix had "failed" or was deemed "incompetent,"[9] and I had to terminate the pregnancy because my amniotic fluid had become infected from my cervix opening too early. In the midst of our devastation, we not only had to navigate the pain of losing two children but had to suffer the indignity of being treated as if their lives didn't matter and neither did ours. We were told of the need to terminate in a sharp, cold sentence from the attending doctor (who was accompanied by medical students shadowing him for training). My mind goes to Pauline Breedlove of Toni Morrison's *The Bluest Eye*, who, while giving birth to Pecola, is visited by a doctor and his shadowing medical students; the doctor proclaims to the group that Black women like Pauline give birth right away with no pain, "just like horses." While the doctor assigned to me didn't say these words, I felt a deep sense of disregard for my physical and emotional pain among most of the various medical providers cycling in and out of my hospital room. In fact, they didn't even notify me about when someone would come in to take me to deliver what would be a stillbirth, so I spent a full day in tears and terror every time a door would open and close—each time thinking they would be coming for the twins. Providers' disregard for the magnitude of my loss and the coldness of the treatment I received amplified the anxiety that I had already been dealing with about becoming a mother because of how Black children are treated in this world. I definitely wanted children, but I wasn't blind to the anti-Blackness of the world I was bringing them into. The disregard for their deaths by the doctors who interacted with me felt like a double injury because of how Black life is devalued. After I was discharged, I replayed the experience over and over in my mind. Where had I gone wrong? Why had no one detected this potential issue? I thought about the large practice where I had received care and the reality that none of them really knew me. In fact, after my loss, during my first visit back to the practice, someone, who hadn't read my chart, asked me about my pregnancy and assumed that since I had delivered them the children were living. I had to announce on multiple occasions that my children were dead.

Also, there were few people I could speak to about my pain. Although miscarriage and stillbirth are more common than many realize, hardly anyone really talks about the experience openly. For some, this is due to the overwhelming nature of the loss. For others it is due to shame or feelings of failure. Because I was studying for my oral exams, I inevitably turned to books to find comfort. I had been reading Toni Morrison's *Beloved* in the lead-up to my medical emergency. I had the novel with me in my bag when I was rushed to the hospital once it was discovered that my cervix had prematurely opened. I had read the novel a couple of times, but when I arrived home after losing my twins, I pulled it out and continued rereading it. The meaning this time around felt especially heavy for me. Here I was in recovery from losing what were my "best things," as Sethe from *Beloved* would say—having to work through cycles of grief and guilt all at the same time. Sethe became a traveling companion for me, and that was when I realized that stories would save me. I went on to get pregnant again, this time with a single pregnancy, a girl that we would name Zoe. She came early as well, but I was far enough along that she could survive outside the womb and in the NICU. I had developed eclampsia with her and nearly died during her birth from seizures. I couldn't help but think about the statistics on higher blood pressure and higher stress levels among Black women, as I had lived in fear of and worked desperately not to have another loss. Ours was a long journey of three months in the hospital with many death scares and traumatic moments. I was told by one of my doctors that my body just could not bear children and that I should get a hysterectomy. That advice landed on me like a ton of bricks. Here I had grown up in the land of Fannie Lou Hamer, a victim of the "Mississippi Appendectomy,"[10] sterilized without her knowledge, and I was being told that I shouldn't have children. I couldn't divorce all I was experiencing in my motherhood journey from the histories that inform how Black women are treated in health care. I refused the sterilization and went on to deliver another child—this time a boy that we would name Jackson. He came full term and healthy. But by that time, I had so much unhealed trauma that mothering without fear had become nearly impossible for me. I sought therapy and other forms of support. I even made the subject of the Black female body in pain the focus of my dissertation. All my subsequent scholarly writing would be informed by Black body politics. My first book, *Staging Black Fugitivity*, explores how the Black body in performance serves as a tool for representing the contemporary resonance of slavery, especially in terms of the ineffability of Black pain. Even as this work was and is necessary, I was writing around my pain. I wanted desperately to tell the story of my birthing experiences somewhere, but I wanted to do so safely and in community. I realized that those kinds of spaces were rare if not nonexistent. I wanted to share space with Black birthing people navigating the devastating statistics on Black maternal mortality. I had nearly lost my life while giving birth and could have easily been a statistic. Survival, however, was not enough. I wanted to *heal*, and I knew I had to do that in community.

BIRTHING THE LIVABLE BLACK FUTURES STORYTELLING PROJECT

Thankfully, I received the opportunity to explore storywork, healing, and reproductive justice through a research grant awarded to me in 2021 from the American Council of Learned Societies to address the ways Black patient voices were left out of conversations about Black sexual and reproductive health, although they were at the center of the harm experienced in medical spaces, and although they carried deep embodied knowledge that could help us truly address the issues we faced. Under the leadership of executive director Marsha Jones, we assembled an amazing team of doulas, advocates, and researchers (D'Andra Willis, Qiana Lewis-Arnold, Helen Zimba, Cerita Burrell, and Dr. Allison Tomlinson) with the goal of advancing conversations about Black sexual and reproductive health, which were critical for the precarious times we were living in. It was within this beloved community that we cocreated the Livable Black Futures Storytelling Project, where we addressed everything from gynecological and obstetric harm to the attacks on bodily autonomy at the state and national levels as this project was carried out in the lead-up to the *Dobbs v. Jackson* decision. Thinking together with Audre Lorde, who writes in "Man Child: A Black Lesbian Feminist's Response," as a Black woman committed to a livable future, "I must examine all my possibilities of being within such a destructive system,"[11] we explored this key question: In naming our experiences of obstetric violence and institutional and medical racism, how can we imagine new possibilities of being and care that enable Black futures?

Given all of the political and social upheaval we were navigating, this project served simultaneously as a practice of memory and of healing. Participants (who will heretofore be referred to as "storytellers" to signal their role as partners with us in creating knowledge and healing in community) were asked to remember things like their first encounters with gynecological medicine, their experiences in medical spaces, and the various traumas that came along with those experiences. They were also asked to imagine new possibilities: What could patient-centered health care look like? What could gynecological and obstetric medicine actually do when engaged through a reproductive justice lens? What ancestral knowledges could be integrated into medical practice? These and more were the substance of our conversations. And much like Morrison's descriptor of writing and the Black imagination in her essay "The Site of Memory," the storytellers' stories often materialized like a flood. Silenced for so long (whether because of shame or the devaluing of their voices), the storytellers broke open the dam between their experiences and the public discourse and released their pain, their trauma, and their joy in shared space.

Eesha Pandit offers up the metaphor that "movements for social justice are rivers."[12] I extend this metaphor to claim that Black storytelling for reproductive justice is a force that is key to moving this work forward. Just as Loretta Ross and Rickie Solinger argue in *Reproductive Justice: An Introduction*, storytelling in reproductive justice is key as a form of resistance and an embrace of polyvocality that shapes the discourse and activates change.[13] It is a mobilizing and community-building force that is both a release and a form of imagining otherwise. Moreover, in *Telling Stories to Change the World*, Rickie Solinger, Madeline Fox, and Kayhan Irani make clear that narrative is a crucial vehicle for reawakening, sharing, and sustaining social justice impulses. Marsha Jones, executive director of the Afiya Center, makes plain the archival and healing power of storytelling. She says:

> And because we stopped telling stories [from shame and other forms of silencing] we had this huge gap [in our historical accounts]—Black folk been catching babies. Black folk been doing abortion. Black folk been healing outside of a doctor's office. Black folk been doing this, but we stopped talking about it. So to start telling stories again and to share stories, that's what's going to heal our nation. That's going to heal our people.

Jones highlights the consequences of the move away from oral traditions in favor of the written word. In the medicalization of childbirth and the virtual disappearance of granny midwives as a result, much of the folk wisdom once shared in community is increasingly less prominent. This is the reality that Marsha Jones laments. Together with Jones, our Livable Black Futures team adopted as the central goal of our research the use of storytelling circles to realize the full power of storywork.[14]

Integrating a literary dimension was key for me because Black women fiction writers have so beautifully narrativized Black birthing people's sexual and reproductive health journeys, utilizing the imagination to direct us toward alternative worlds. However, this kind of formal storytelling is often treated separately from the kinds of storytelling that work in the service of social justice or the stories gained in settings like focus groups. Works such as Toni Morrison's *Beloved* and *The Bluest Eye*, Gayl Jones's *Corregidora*, Dolen Perkins-Valdez's *Take My Hand*, Octavia Butler's *Parable of the Sower*, and Jamaica Kincaid's *The Autobiography of My Mother* serve as what I call the *imaginative and narrative arm* of reproductive justice. This is also true for Black women poets such as Lucille Clifton and Audre Lorde, as well as playwrights such as Lorraine Hansberry (*A Raisin in the Sun*) and Anyika McMillan Herod (*Do No Harm*). Their work adds a deeper level of analysis into the inner lives of Black women experiencing gynecological and obstetric violence. I was particularly taken by Dána-Ain Davis's *Reproductive Injustice*, which begins each chapter with the voice of a Black woman writer. She intertwines the creative work of Black women with her exploration of Black women's experiences in neonatal intensive care units and how what she terms *reproductive injustice* shapes their experiences. Using the imaginative and narrative work of Black feminist creatives, *We Are Pregnant with Freedom* aims to probe the intersections between the storytelling work conducted in focus groups and interviews and the imaginative work of Black birthing people, as well as to examine how these narratives work together in the service of reproductive justice. In this work, we use Black feminist creative writing as models of breaking silences about issues in sexual and reproductive health that are often stigmatized and as texts that offer insight into the inner lives of Black birthing people's journeys regarding sexual and reproductive health in ways no other discourse has offered. These works became and remain key to our methodology of using story to engender more stories. Or as Byllye Avery so compellingly states, "When women make their stories public, without the shame and embarrassment that keep us silent about our health, we become active participants in our health, and those who listen to them and support them benefit as well."[15] Our storytelling method was based on the hypothesis that stories beget more stories, that they become generative sources of knowledge and inspiration that enable Black women and birthing people to be authors of their own experiences and healing.

S.R. Toliver's *Recovering Black Storytelling in Qualitative Research: Endarkened Storywork* also represents the kind of scholarly inquiry that is at the heart of this book. Wanting to move away from academics being considered singularly as the collectors of tales, she aims to show how Black researchers also inherit a long tradition of Black storywork that informs their own intellectual and creative production. She explains,

> Ultimately, *Endarkened Storywork* is one way of showing we are serious enough—dedicated enough—to making space for other ways of thinking, knowing, interpreting, and representing our work. It centers community by relying on communal ways of being and knowing rather than committing to becoming the autonomous individual uplifted by the enlightenment. It remembers responsibility by forcing us to interrogate our writing and consider how it aligns with or against methods used by the communities we are blessed to work with.[16]

Toliver highlights how storywork shifts ideological understandings of knowledge making and who can be considered experts. My work in amplifying Black feminist storytelling is animated by a similar desire to center communal knowledges, especially those that are often marginalized. This posture also signals the need to hold in tension one's role in the academy, where researchers have often gone into communities and caused harm, and one's Black identity, which cannot be divorced from the research. Eschewing myths of objectivity and Western ways of knowing, Toliver espouses an ethic that aligns with the work I aimed to do with my partners at the Afiya Center and with our research participants more broadly. I knew that I could not feign objectivity or divorce myself from the cultural experiences that shaped who I was and that I brought to bear on my work, so I took on a posture of participant-researcher, being clear with our storytellers that this was as much a personal inquiry as an academic one. If the academy could be enlightened by the knowledge produced in this space, I welcomed it, but my central goal was (and remains) to create a safe and supportive space for Black birthing people to speak about their experiences so that their knowledges can be lifted up and utilized to improve the lives of all birthing people and to do so alongside them. I had seen many articles about the Black maternal mortality crisis, and I was glad to see people writing about these issues. However, most of the perspectives came from medical professionals and researchers who were not Black birthing people. Moreover, many of them resorted to patient blame,[17] claiming that if Black birthing people would only lose weight, stop smoking, and see their doctors more (never mind if they lived far away from doctors or didn't have sufficient medical insurance for such visits), they would survive. I also saw little to no discussion about Black birthing people who were queer, gender nonbinary, disabled, weight stigmatized, incarcerated, or living with HIV. These are marginalized identities in medicine and medical research, but just like heteronormative birthing people, they see gynecologists, and they give birth, so we have to account for their experiences as well.

This book aims to engage with and amplify the stories of what I term *Black gynecological publics*, which I locate in writing, in organizing work, and through focus groups—publics that are emerging as the reproductive justice movement evolves. These storytellers enter the space made possible by reproductive justice theorizing that centers itself on human rights and goes beyond matters of reproduction. Additionally, they illuminate what it means to sustain life in an ethical and just way. Their collective public storytelling serves as a means of healing and community building. These Black gynecological publics also enable confrontations with historical erasures and the legacies of those histories. As Monica McLemore and Esther Choo make plain, "When community voices are missing, accountability and transparency are impossible to achieve."[18] *We Are Pregnant with Freedom* asserts that community is central to repair and collective liberation. In doing so, it traces *Black sexual and reproductive liberation narratives*, my term that situates such storywork in the tradition of the Black radical imagination across time from slave narratives to the present. These narratives map out various paths to freedom in this precarious time. Holistically, this book charts genealogies of experience as well as new forms of advocacy that can serve as guides for future generations.

The advancement of Black sexual and reproductive liberation narratives not only offers methodologies for enacting bodily autonomy and freedom but also produces a cleansing of the mind and spirit in the face of oppression. The waters of Black communities in the United States have experienced varying degrees of deadly contamination: Belews Lake in North Carolina, frequented by Black residents, polluted with coal ash from Duke Energy;[19]

Flint, Michigan, a largely Black city that still contends with an ongoing crisis of lead in the water supply;[20] Jackson, Mississippi, another largely Black city that frequently experiences such instability in the water supply that in many cases the city has lacked potable water for months, causing school closures and health crises;[21] Hurricane Katrina, which produced a deadly flood of water into the predominantly Black Ninth Ward of New Orleans.[22] These are but a few instances where we see blackness and water intertwined, often in precarious ways.

And yes, there is the life-giving force of waterbreaking as a form of the body's preparation for childbirth. It often happens unexpectedly, and the rush sets off a scurrying of support to bring a new baby into the world, but this is not a universal experience, especially now that modern medicine is more intertwined with childbirth, often disrupting natural processes of pregnancy and delivery. Cesarean sections predominate in childbirth practices (especially for Black birthing people) to such an extent that there are efforts to address the frequency.[23] Although I've been pregnant three times, my water never broke of its own volition. In my first pregnancy, when I was induced because of an unviable pregnancy, my water was broken for me, and in the subsequent ones this process was circumvented because of unplanned and planned cesarean sections.

I think on this and the relationship between water and Black storytelling, and it sheds some light on why it took me over twelve years to find the words for my experience. The denied release, both mental and physical, that I experienced constituted a rupture of my bodymind, and I had to intentionally put myself back together. In the Livable Black Futures Storytelling Project, we had storytellers in similar states of being who were sharing their stories for the first time (for some, many years after the initial experience). And with each meeting, I felt the accumulating force of our stories coming together, combining with histories of oppression Black birthing people have faced (from forced pregnancy to forced sterilization and more). I think of us as creating and experiencing a palimpsest of stories layered one on top of the other, but I also see these stories as a form of flooding, of collective waterbreaking.

It is a breaking of silence.
It is movement.
It is a flood.
It is tears.
It is rain.
It is a cleansing, a healing, a life giving.
It is making space for freedom.

We can think of *waterbreaking* as the outpouring of story from those who have experienced silencing and being unheard due to marginalization of various kinds. The sharing of these suppressed narratives makes space for creativity, exploration, and healing.

WE ARE PREGNANT WITH FREEDOM

The line that inspires this book's title, "We are pregnant with freedom," comes from Assata Shakur's political autobiography, *Assata*. In it, she details her political prosecution for her alleged involvement in the death of a New Jersey state trooper in 1973. A member of the Black Panther Party and later the Black Liberation Army, Shakur was a target of the state, resulting in numerous prosecutions and her ultimate relocation to Cuba, where she currently lives in asylum from US political persecution. Shakur's autobiography not only details the brutality she endured in the New Jersey and New York penal system but also describes her experience conceiving and giving birth to her only daughter, Kakuya, while incarcerated. She became pregnant with Kakuya while on trial with her comrade Kamau Sadiki for a 1972 Bronx bank robbery. They were held together away from the courtroom, and during this time they contemplated many facets of their futures. Seeing the bleak realities of their incarceration, they made the conscious decision to conceive as a way to resist the state's efforts to control their fates. For Assata, birthing was deeply political. She states, "I'm going to live as hard as I can and as full as I can until I die. And I'm not letting the parasites, these oppressors, these greedy racist swine make me kill my children in my mind, before they are even born."[24] Assata's words speak to the complexity of reproductive justice. More than just a matter of having access to abortion, the framework equally speaks to the right to have a child, something Black women have had to fight for since slavery. The right to mother, to have children and to parent them in safe and healthy communities, is often a chief concern alongside abortion rights. This is why it is key to complicate conversations on reproductive justice beyond abortion.

For Assata, having children served as an expression of love and community. This radical choice was a way to mitigate the despair of surviving in a deeply anti-Black world. Assata affirmed that love is central to liberation. After she decided to get pregnant, she penned the poem "Love," which reads:

> Love is a contraband in Hell,
> cause love is acid
> that eats away bars.

> But you, me, and tomorrow
> hold hands and make vows
> that struggle will multiply.
>
> The hacksaw has two blades.
>
> The shotgun has two barrels.
>
> We are pregnant with freedom.
>
> We are a conspiracy.[25]

This poem speaks so much to what reproductive justice is about. With the increasing encroachment of the carceral state into various institutions (medical, educational, financial, and more), Assata's experience becomes salient for conversations about bodily autonomy and injustice. The prison is a key site where we can see what Saidiya Hartman aptly names the "afterlives of slavery": "skewed life chances, limited access to health and education, premature death, incarceration, and impoverishment."[26] Reproductive justice won't be realized until we address what is happening in our prisons, especially when it comes to health care delivery. For Assata Shakur to dream about freedom and love amid the dire circumstances she faced represents an ultimate form of resistance. She gives language to collective struggle for reproductive justice and more. This is why "We are pregnant with freedom" resonated so powerfully with me as the title of this book. I want to have a conversation not just about reproduction but about what radical movements for reproductive justice give birth to, whether one has had children or not. We are all implicated in this work.

While I will expand more on *Assata* in my chapter on carcerality, abolition medicine, and sexual and reproductive health, it is key here to discuss how her autobiography serves as an intellectual apparatus for the book. With its blend of creative and imaginative storytelling alongside illuminating accounts of life in prison and her coming of age in the mid-twentieth century, *Assata* is a representation of the kinds of work I aim to collectivize in this book: the testimonies, the poetry, the songs, the journals, the conversations, the wails, and more.

Moreover, *Assata* offers a guide for scholars who are working in community for justice. Assata states that when she was contemplating going back to college, she didn't want to be an intellectual, spending most of her time in libraries and disengaged from what was happening on the streets. She says, "Theory without practice is just as incomplete as practice without theory. The two have to go together."[27] These words guided my approach to moving my previous work in literary analyses of Black narratives engaging with reproductive justice to a more tangible connection between imaginative work and its impact on people's lives. Along with S.R. Toliver's use of "endarkened storywork" to offer alternative representations of data that are better attuned to Black storytelling praxes, Venus Evans-Winters's *Black Feminism in Qualitative Inquiry* provided a road map for how I might do this. Winters uses the metaphor of the mosaic, an art form that is the product of diverse elements, patterns, and forms (much like Black quilt-making and collage traditions), to describe and enact a race- and gender-based approach to qualitative inquiry and analysis. Rather than offer homogeneous representations of Black experience in her work, she draws on this mosaic because it "brings forth an aesthetically distinct alternative to widely accepted notions of how knowledge production and acquisition should transpire in qualitative inquiry and analysis."[28] Aligning with this approach was key for me because my work aimed to gather a broad array of Black birthing people and experiences. I knew I would need to rely on methods that were nontraditional and, in many ways, experimental.

ON METHOD

This book relies on a mosaic of approaches and principles of tracing and analyzing Black storywork that follows in the tradition of the Black radical imagination. The aforementioned S.R. Toliver and Venus Evans-Winters are foundational for me, but I am also thinking with theorists within the Black literary tradition. Toni Morrison, who opens this introduction, has always been a North Star in my analytical work. Her description of the "site of memory" as a space of embodied history and her articulation of a practice of "literary archaeology"[29] that brings forward the voices of silenced Black people in the archive offer a way for me to engage with this work through lenses of memory and history. Across this book, I explore the histories and contemporary experiences of Black birthing people through the metaphor of a palimpsest, a mosaic layering of stories of embodied histories and the living out of the implications of those histories. Additionally, Saidiya Hartman's method of critical fabulation, which she uses to represent Black people in the archive from slavery to the early twentieth century, is a practice of narrative restraint—of letting the subaltern speak, as Gayatri Spivak would have it.[30] It is an attempt to recover an unrecoverable past; "It is a narrative of what might have been or could have been; it is a history written with and against the archive."[31] Hartman's approach can be extended to think about the contemporary silences in archival spaces like hospital medical records. Within that institutional archive, the patient's voice is largely absent. Medical historians like

Deirdre Cooper Owens and Harriet Washington offer us a window into what it means to interrogate the medical archive.[32] Through work such as this we see how Black feminist storytelling for reproductive justice can shed new light on histories and beget other stories.

My work is largely in the service of attending to those who have experienced harm in the present but have limited outlets to tell their version of events. Through having the Livable Black Futures storytellers engage in creative expression, I aimed to enable them to return to their experiences and break their own silences. It was a form of critical fabulation that was self-guided. In creatively exploring their own unspeakable experiences, they drew on the power to name the experiences and understand them better with Hartman's words in mind: "The necessity of trying to represent what we cannot, rather than leading to pessimism or despair must be embraced as the impossibility that conditions our knowledge of the past and animates our desire for a liberated future."[33] I embraced the challenge of exploring our pasts and the archive of painful memory as a way to move toward our collective goal of imagining and ultimately enacting a liberated future—a livable Black future. Not only did Audre Lorde's "Man Child" provide the language of the notion of a livable Black future (as stated above), but engaging with this 1979 essay in 2020 in advance of this project also served as a stark reminder that her concerns about the futurity of Black children still remain. They are still growing up in a hostile, anti-Black, and sexist world, and it is imperative to imagine ways of surviving in these contexts and creating the world we want to see.

This book is concerned with Black storytelling for reproductive justice as a means to trace a tradition and speak to the ongoing ways storytelling is needed for those situated at the perilous intersections of the contemporary realities of police violence, mass incarceration, HIV, anti-Blackness, queer phobia, antiabortion efforts, the maternal mortality and Covid mortality crises, and more. I use storytelling as a path to reproductive and sexual freedom with the salient words of the 1977 Combahee River Collective in mind: "If Black women were free, it would mean that everyone else would have to be free since our freedom would necessitate the destruction of all the systems of oppression."[34] The writers center Black women in this conversation as a way to illuminate the intersecting oppressions that converge on Black women—those who inhabit multiply marginalized identities and who are often the most affected by varying forms of oppression. Yet their voices are often deemphasized in favor of those with more resources and access. This is also a motivating idea behind the work of the twelve Black women (known as the Women of African Descent for Reproductive Justice) who created the concept of reproductive justice in 1994 at a conference sponsored by the Illinois Pro-Choice Alliance and the Ms. Foundation for Women in Chicago. At the conference, these Black women intervened in conversations that prioritized the abortion binary without regard for what happens to vulnerable birthing people before, during, and after pregnancies. Loretta Ross explains, "When we centered ourselves in our lens, we understood how intersectional paradigms could reframe historical inequalities and differences in power and opportunities that affect our reproductive behaviors. Rather than accommodating ourselves in a pro-choice paradigm, we chose to transform the model itself."[35] They knew that this model would offer a more expansive vision of reproductive justice for all. Considering how Black feminist thought and Black birthing people are at the heart of this work, I wanted to center Black storytelling as a companion to transforming the conversations we have about reproductive justice beyond the abortion binary. It is my deeply held belief that achieving reproductive justice and fully realizing its goals requires centering the voices of Black birthing people (particularly those with multiply marginalized identities) because doing so necessitates a reckoning with oppressive systems that maintain systemic health and social inequalities.

Our cocreated methodology for the Livable Black Futures Storytelling Project was rooted in key ethics of care, safety, creating an environment free of shame and stigma, and giving our storytellers the support and tools to fully show up unapologetically in the space (whether in person or virtual). We began with the philosophy that Black birthing people were worthy of financial investment and support. Therefore, we paid our storytellers an amount that would appropriately compensate them for their time without being coercive. We provided childcare services and dinners so that these after-work needs would not be a barrier to participation. We enacted care through providing stress balls and fidget toys when conversations became challenging, and we provided art-making opportunities to work through ways to represent inexpressible painful experiences. Moreover, we approached this work as participant-researchers, refusing the myth of objectivity and the notion of knowledge hierarchies. We worked actively to remind the storytellers of their embodied knowledges and their voices as equally valid in conversations on how to address the health challenges facing Black birthing people. Importantly, we worked to make the space inclusive with respect to sexuality, access to resources, and other factors that often limit participants from engagement. Prioritizing inclusivity created a space where people who were gender-queer, nonbinary, lesbian, formerly incarcerated, living with HIV, underresourced, and more would feel supported and heard. In the process, group members learned a great deal from one another and expanded our conceptions of just who conversations about sexual and reproductive health are for. A central point of pride from this work was that we were able to form a supportive and inclusive space where Black birthing people could feel empowered to speak about all the ways they had experienced harm in terms of their sexual and reproductive health. Last, I want to note that I use pseudonyms for the storytellers in our research work to protect their identities while affirming their humanity.

WHERE THIS BOOK ENTERS

We Are Pregnant with Freedom benefits from key scholarship that focuses on the experiences of Black birthing people and the fight for reproductive justice. The writing and activism of thinkers such as Loretta Ross, Rickie Solinger, Byllye Avery, and Marsha Jones ground me in my understanding of the critical importance of storytelling for reproductive justice. Additionally, the following monographs have been foundational to shaping my approach. Dorothy Roberts's *Killing the Black Body* provides key histories of the ways Black reproduction has been a target of state violence and injustice. Khiara Bridges's *Reproducing Race* shows, through ethnography in a New York City public hospital, the ways that racialization in medicine has dire consequences for birthing people of color, particularly for those who are economically vulnerable. Dána Ain Davis's *Reproductive Injustice* explores the ways medical racism affects the experiences of Black birthing people who have given birth to premature and low-birth-weight infants. Deirdre Cooper Owens's *Medical Bondage* offers a historical account of how gynecological medicine was forged on the bodies of enslaved Black women who were considered "medical superbodies," ripe for experimentation and exploitation. These works provided me with key frameworks to explore the ways medical racism and mistreatment still shape the experiences of Black birthing people. Scholars such as Monica McLemore, Esther Choo, Karen Scott, Joia Crear-Perry, and Linda Villarosa set forth key concepts such as obstetric racism, social and structural determinants of health, eugenics in medicine, and more to effectively name the sources of harm that Black birthing people experience.

Recently, scholarship has emerged that seeks to expand just who is included in these conversations and to explore how we can achieve reproductive justice for all. Alexis Pauline Gumbs, China Martens, and Ma'ia Williams's *Revolutionary Mothering* centers marginalized mothers of color, including queer mothers, to show how they create powerful visions of the future while navigating a precarious present. Dani McClain's *We Live for the We* highlights how Black mothers in our present era deal with the ongoing police violence that gets spectacularized on our screens. She traces mothers working in movements for social, political, and cultural change to address these issues. Jennifer Nash argues in *Birthing Black Mothers* that although Black motherhood as a political category has often rendered Black mothers as flattened figures identified only through loss, Black mothers are transforming the concept and culturally representing and theorizing new modes of Black motherhood. Most recently, Cara Page and Ericka Woodland have offered the collection *Healing Justice Lineages*, which explores the history, legacies, and liberatory practices of healing justice—a political strategy of collective and community care and safety that intervenes in generational trauma from systemic violence and oppression. Nessette Falu's *Unseen Flesh* considers the experiences of Black lesbians in Brazil and their encounters with medical bias as well as how they engage in resistance and abolitionist practices of worth making that sustain Black queer identity and living. Finally, Janet Garcia-Hallett's *Invisible Mothers* explores the experiences of formerly incarcerated mothers in New York City and the various challenges of reentry due to patriarchy, misogyny, and systemic racism.

Taken together, these studies lay the groundwork for *We Are Pregnant with Freedom*. They take up various efforts of Black birthing people to achieve reproductive justice. *We Are Pregnant with Freedom* adds to this discourse by centering Black feminist storytelling and Black radical imagination as key to the work of reproductive justice. It advances multiple analytics from Black feminist qualitative research to literary and narrative analysis in order to raise up key voices and conversations taking place in our present vexing moment.

HOW THIS BOOK IS STRUCTURED

This book traces my journey to engage the many valences of Black feminist storytelling for reproductive justice, primarily across the years of 2020–22. It is a blend of literary analysis and qualitative engagement with the stories of the Livable Black Futures Project as well as those offered by scholars and other theorists in efforts to advance reproductive justice. Essentially, it is a collection of the critical narrative work of the emerging Black gynecological publics that I trace in the book. I begin each chapter with an affirmation in the spirit of the Livable Black Futures Storytelling Project: we relied on affirmations for strength as we revisited painful experiences and as an articulation of our value. I form my own here in the hopes that the book will reflect the kind of space we worked to create.

Chapter 1, "Toward a Radical *We*: Decolonizing Sexual and Reproductive Health," offers a blend of voices (queer, trans, disabled, weight stigmatized, living with HIV, and more) in order to deepen our conversations on reproductive justice and advance a radical *we* that functions as a site of resistance to heteronormative medicine, which is also at the heart of the Black maternal mortality crisis. I begin the work in this way because these voices are crucial to moving us closer to fully realizing reproductive justice for all. Rather than treat these issues separately, I use an intersectional approach because these identities are seldom separate categories for individuals. This conversation necessarily raises the dynamic of reproductive justice solidarities and the importance of cultivating a movement that affects large groups of people differently positioned in society but sharing common traumas as a result of reproductive oppression and heteropatriarchal white supremacy. These groups experience challenges mobilizing across difference: for example, some participants are entirely focused on the issue of abortion even though reproductive justice is much more expansive than that, and others would fall into the category of TERFs (trans-exclusionary feminists, i.e., cisgender women who are hostile to transwomen).[36]

Chapter 2, "Reproductive Justice: An American Grammar," is a collection of key terms that I use in the book, including ones that serve as important supplemental information for exploring the subject matter in the book in deeper ways. You might decide to read this section first, before exploring the rest of the book, or you might read it between chapters, selecting terms that feel relevant to the chapter with which you are engaged. As some might say, "Choose your own adventure." This chapter catalogs the terms that marginalized Black birthing people use, as well as key terms used in relation to reproductive justice. It is influenced by thinkers such as Hortense Spillers and Christina Sharpe, who encourage us to interrogate language and construct new grammars to more efficiently talk and think about the complexities of Black experience. In doing so, this work gathers key terms for the conversations informing this book and broader discussions about reproductive justice. While not fully comprehensive, it maps out the key ideas animating this work. It is my goal that this grammar becomes a tool for teaching and thinking about reproductive justice. It is important to note that I use both the term *women* and the term *birthing people* to offer an expansive framing that includes those who identify as women as well as those who are not binary or queer yet are also subject to gynecological and obstetric medicine.

Chapter 3, "Rememory: A Reproductive Justice Mixtape," offers insight into the structure of the Livable Black Futures Project and explores foundational narratives produced by Black artists in the service of reproductive justice. I examine the *Mothers of Gynecology* statues of Montgomery, Alabama, artist Michelle Browder as well as the music of artists such as Megan Thee Stallion and the poetry of reelaviolette botts-ward. The chapter contemplates the significance of this artistry as an ongoing space of creative intervention into the challenges facing Black birthing people or even as a creative form of sexual and reproductive liberation. In this work we can see otherwise imagining and the life-giving force of creativity. In many ways, this chapter is offered as a mixtape—an exploration of various forms of creative work in the service of bodily liberation and justice.

In keeping with the theme of the power of Black imaginative work, chapter 4, "Imagining Livable Black Futures," looks at how stories engender other stories. This chapter draws on the work of thinkers such as Audre Lorde, Robin D.G. Kelley, Octavia Butler, and adrienne maree brown, as well as the knowledge producers of the Livable Black Futures Storytelling Project, to see how Black storytelling for reproductive justice pushes us forward—from our precarious present to an otherwise imagining that can facilitate community building and the cocreation of our futures. This work serves as a form of strategizing in oppressive times. Envisioning future possibilities offers us paths to surviving and thriving in our present and beyond. Reproductive justice is animated by freedom dreams and is a key example of this concept at work.

Chapter 5, "Abolition Medicine," moves to those who often exist on the margins of the margins, namely those who experience carceral medicine. This chapter raises up the full subjectivities of Black birthing people who have experienced incarceration. It is an account of my engagement with this community in Dallas, Texas, via our storytelling project. Alongside their stories, I examine the more public accounts of Assata Shakur and her political autobiography, *Assata*, as well as the visual artistry of Mary Enoch Elizabeth Baxter (aka Isis Tha Savior) and her account of giving birth while imprisoned in her song and art installation *Ain't I a Woman*. Collectively, these stories offer a narrative and visual dimension to the inhumane treatment of Black birthing people in prisons, including shackling while giving birth, poor medical care, and immediate child separation—thereby producing rippling traumatic effects. It is key to engage with carcerality when considering reproductive justice because every modern-day indignity that comes from the denial of reproductive autonomy can be found in incarcerated women's lives.

Chapter 6, "Policing Black Birth," continues the conversation about policing Black birthing people and by extension Black families. Utilizing Christina Sharpe's framework of "the weather," which she defines as the totalizing environment of anti-Blackness,

I examine how this anti-Black weather shapes the birthing process for Black birthing people, sometimes resulting in family separation. Correspondingly, I consider the various forms of storytelling that Black mothers and families are using to highlight the harms they experience from family policing, particularly while pregnant and during or immediately after having given birth. In the narratives I trace, we can see Black mothers still fighting for legitimacy in a deeply anti-Black world. Their stories constitute a disruption of prevailing controlling images of Black motherhood and shed light on the harms of family policing and separation, a key conversation that needs amplification in reproductive justice work, as scholars such as Dorothy Roberts remind us.

I conclude with a meditation on the time period that closes the span of the storytelling research project—June 2022. During this period, *Dobbs v. Jackson Women's Health Organization* was decided by the US Supreme Court and ultimately took away the constitutional right to an abortion. I document what it has meant to live in Texas, where trigger laws (an apt name because of their deadly implications) to effectively ban abortion have taken effect, and what that means for this work. Even though reproductive justice is about much more than abortion rights, the denial of bodily autonomy and reproductive freedom has direct implications for Black women and birthing people and is drawn from a long history of unfreedom surrounding Black birth. In this chapter, I contemplate Assata Shakur's writing. Even though she was writing while imprisoned, the motivations driving her work resonate because of the precarious situation (and unlivable living—to call up Treva Lindsey)[37] of Black birthing people in the present. Assata Shakur's words call to us today. How will our stories, our collectivity, and our advocacy help us get free?

It is my desire that *We Are Pregnant with Freedom: Black Feminist Storytelling for Reproductive Justice* breaks through the barriers to unapologetic Black storytelling (whether issues of access, shame, stigma, or a general disregard for the voices of multiply marginalized folks). I also aim to advance possibilities for raising up the voices of Black birthing people by offering my own methodology and process as a path to do this work. Continuing with my concept of waterbreaking, I want this book to facilitate conversations where such a process can continue to occur beyond this book. In Toni Morrison's *Beloved*, when the character Beloved (a representation of Sethe's dead child) shows up unexpectedly, having just walked out of the water while fully dressed, Sethe experiences a sudden need to void water herself. She attempts to stop the voiding, "But there was no stopping water breaking from a breaking womb and there was no stopping it now."[38] Although Sethe is not pregnant at this time, the seeming return of the daughter that she killed to avoid her growing up enslaved causes a flooding of water, a breaking that creates space for her to reckon with her past and heal from it. That flooding is a force that no one can stop. It is what I think of when I consider the stories that flow from this book. Like social justice movements, they are rivers that build power from their collective force. Let the waterbreaking that I trace in this book birth new stories and strengthen our resolve to fight for change.

CHAPTER ONE

Toward a Radical *We*

Decolonizing Sexual and Reproductive Health

Affirmation
I claim my right to care that affirms my dignity. I deserve care that is free from ableism, transphobia, homophobia, fatphobia, and shame.

In 2019, when I began focused research on Black stories that dealt with issues of Black maternal mortality as well as sexual and reproductive health more broadly, I was troubled to see a preponderance of stories that centered a relatively narrow profile of Black mothers or victims of Black maternal mortality. They were usually middle class, college educated, nondisabled, cisgendered women. Many of these women were like me, and I certainly saw a good deal of my story in them. I mourned their experiences alongside my own. Yet I couldn't escape the fact that essentially, these stories aligned with the perpetuation of "perfect victim narratives," which are often used as a way to garner public support around an injustice—holding up someone who wasn't supposed to die. In reality, no one should die in childbirth or experience any form of medical racism/harm, yet we rarely see or hear stories of the different groups of people implicated in gynecological and obstetric medicine whose lives are equally at risk when it comes to surviving pregnancy and childbirth. Because they occupy positionalities from being queer to being disabled to living with HIV and more, they are often relegated to the *margins of the margins* in conversations about Black maternal/perinatal health. Moreover, I found that the discourse largely excluded conversations about the broader impact of gynecological health care, which is rooted in heteronormativity and often serves as a precursor to obstetric discrimination in medicine. This is where critical work is needed in reproductive justice research. Reproductive justice work is premised on the belief that all people deserve to give birth and parent in safe and healthy environments, and many reproductive justice organizations are working toward just that. Yet the discourse places limits on just which people are foregrounded or even mentioned in this advocacy work. This is why my research on Black feminist storytelling for reproductive justice could not be framed or primarily informed by the mainstream narratives I was encountering. I needed to amplify the experiences of those who aren't always centered. Tien Sydnor-Campbell is instructive on the urgency of greater inclusion in sexual and reproductive health research. Thinking with Valerie Purdie-Vaughns and Richard P. Eibach, Sydnor-Campbell examines the notion of "intersectional invisibility" and how heterocentrism, androcentrism, and ethnocentrism in medicine often invisibilize people who don't fit neatly into racial, gender, and ethnic categories.[1] She cites Black disabled women as a population deeply affected by intersectional invisibility. In many ways, intersectional invisibility is an apt explanation for the limited data and public discourse on the sexual and reproductive health experiences of those who inhabit complex social identities (e.g., queer, incarcerated, weight-stigmatized, disabled). For these reasons, I knew that if I were to truly enact a Black feminist method and politics in my research, my work had to reflect all those affected, especially those who are most vulnerable and often most stigmatized. We can never fully address the Black maternal health crisis or issues of obstetric violence/medical racism without their stories.

This chapter brings forward *Black gynecological publics*, a diverse collective of voices articulating a Black feminist ethic of reproductive justice that is fully inclusive and invested in advancing an anticolonial approach to medicine that addresses historical and ongoing harm. Throughout this book, these voices will play a key role in articulating knowledges and methodologies that advance sexual and reproductive freedom and justice. First, I offer a holistic examination of what it means to decolonize sexual and reproductive health. I then explore the various experiential standpoints (queer, disabled, those living with HIV, and those combating weight stigma) and the unique knowledges they offer. I do not want to suggest that these experiences are distinct from one another, however. It is for this reason that I want to draw attention to what I refer to as *intersectional medical indignity*. This concept names the ways that various biases in medicine can often converge on one body (for instance, if one is Black, disabled, and queer). These voices are crucial to moving us closer to fully realizing reproductive justice for all. This conversation necessarily raises the dynamic of creating reproductive justice solidarities and cultivating a movement that affects large groups of people who, while differently positioned in society, share common traumas as a result of reproductive oppression and heteropatriarchal white supremacy. So I look at the specificity and the intersections of these experiences together. Additionally, I look at the carceral dimensions of this conversation here, but I focus exclusively on carceral medicine in a separate chapter, "Abolition Medicine" (chapter 5). In my research, I found that Black incarcerated women and birthing people are treated as disposable and that their stories can be understood through the continuum of slavery and the treatment of Black bodies as property. Until we address the violence of carceral medicine in prisons and its particular impact on Black birthing people, we can never fully achieve reproductive justice.

Collectively, the voices that this chapter raises up constitute a "radical *we*," a blend of voices that occupy non-normative identities and force us to reckon with and resist the heteronormativity medicine that is also at the heart of the Black maternal mortality crisis. The term *radical we* (with an emphasis on *we*), coined by Marshall Green, resonates deeply with me because it is a way of naming the collectivity of all those implicated in reproductive justice work. Through this radical *we*, we can organize across difference without diluting the specificity of individual experiences. According to Green, "The Black feminist call for an androgynous self is a call to recognize the *them/we* always present in the I which seemed to be forgotten when all the *women* were thought to be white and all the Blacks were thought to be men in social and political thought and praxis."[2] Black feminist interruptions in these rigid categories open space for a radical *we* to emerge. It is from this position that I situate myself in this work as well as the critical work of this book. It is rooted in the declaration of the Black feminist ancestor with whom I share a Mississippi Delta homeland, Fannie Lou Hamer: none of us are free until everyone is free.[3] It is also the radical *we* that I invoke in the book's title drawn from Assata Shakur's words "We are pregnant with freedom."

This radical *we* brings together all those who are marginalized in the discourse and whose unfreedom necessitates such a radical conception of a new world and destruction of the old one.

DECOLONIZING SEXUAL AND REPRODUCTIVE HEALTH

Black, queer sex educator Ericka Hart offers key insights into what it means to decolonize sexual and reproductive health. A breast cancer survivor and a queer person who has given birth in the medical space, Hart makes clear the ways heteronormativity is infused within medicine. She says we need to decolonize health care in order to create more viable outcomes for marginalized people. She uses her own birth story as an illustration of both the hardships and the possibilities of navigating sexual and reproductive health as a queer person.[4] Her birth story is not one that we typically hear about when we are talking about bias in reproductive health care and its toll on Black birthing people. Yet it mirrors the experiences of many cisgendered Black birthing people who are often centered in broader conversations about obstetric racism and the Black maternal health crisis. Hart developed pre-eclampsia while pregnant with her child, East, and experienced everything from queerphobia to fatphobia as she had to relinquish control over her birthing experience because of the life-threatening complications she faced. She laments that "there are so many people training to be midwives, but so many of them do not have the training on how to support queer and trans folks." What Hart's experience also reveals is how much sexual and reproductive health is shaped by heteronormative and overall normative constructs and how critical it is to address these. Alongside the complications that come with dealing with medical racism as a Black birthing person are additional issues that arise when these statuses are coupled with other marginalizations such as disability, queerness, plus size, or economic insecurity. Often Black birthing people occupy multiple marginalized categories as they seek care. Yet the reporting on the Black maternal health crisis seldom accounts for the complexities of Black birthing people, often favoring flattened, monolithic stories of those affected by obstetric harm. For instance, a July 2023 Reuters article reported recent research findings that the "number of U.S. women who died within a year after pregnancy more than doubled between 1999 and 2019, with the highest deaths among Black women."[5] The article also cited central causes for these deaths as relayed by the US Centers for Disease Control and Prevention. They are mental health conditions, excessive bleeding, cardiac and coronary conditions, infections, blood clots, and pregnancy-related high blood pressure. The unspoken truth regarding these issues is that they align with harmful practices in medicine such as ableism, fatphobia, heteronormativity, and a host of other biases that can influence or exacerbate issues such as high blood pressure, mental health conditions, and cardiac and coronary conditions. Moreover, issues such as blood clots, excessive bleeding, and infections can often be the result of medical neglect.

The report also refers to "Black women" rather than using gender-inclusive terms such as *Black birthing people*, which signify that not all those who give birth are cisgendered women. Organizations and researchers often use this flattening when trying to message a crisis to large swaths of people. The common wisdom is that complexity dilutes the message. But at what cost? Rather than advance reductive and binaristic terminology in sexual and reproductive health, educators like Hart remind us of our responsibility to disrupt these limited frameworks.

The work of Hart and many others challenging the heteronormative logics of medicine is underscored by the movement to decolonize birth led by organizations such as Voices for Birth Justice, the Southern Roots Doula Collective, Black Women's Birth Justice, SisterSong, and more who advocate for full inclusion in birth work regardless of gender or sexuality. Voices for Birth Justice describes their mission as follows: "To challenge systems of oppression, such as racism and sexism in reproductive care, Birth Justice advocates for culturally-appropriate, person-centered care while challenging disrespectful care. It also supports the sharing of knowledge amongst communities and improves access to breastfeeding support and traditional birth-workers, such as midwives and doulas."[6] This includes validation of ancestral knowledges and anticolonial methods of enacting care. Maria Lugones explains in "The Coloniality of Gender" that the cognitive needs of colonialism and capitalism produced ways of knowing that were invested in measurement, quantification, and objectification. These ways of knowing made it possible for colonial and capitalist systems to reconceive the human fictionally in biological terms to form Eurocentric theories of social class—otherwise known as the modern colonial gender system. Moreover, these systems were contingent on eugenics and compulsory heterosexuality, which also served to perpetuate their hierarchies.

Colonial logics show up not only in the delivery of medicine but also in the conducting of research relating to sexual and reproductive health. The authors of "Two Eyed Seeing: Decolonizing Methodologies for Reproductive Justice" note the "inextricable link between colonialism, racism, and reproductive health."[7] They call for new research methods that recognize an array of worldviews as well as research that is informed *by* the community rather than done *for* them. I knew that when I embarked on my own project, I wanted my research to be informed by and accountable to the communities with which I was engaging. I also wanted to center those most affected by these issues. My entry point to this was story. Storywork is key for me because it is within this work that healing can be enacted and narratives shifted. Like S.R. Toliver, I needed to engage in a "deep study of story and consider the multiple ways in which history, community, and self are imbued within Black narratives."[8] This work requires using decolonizing methodologies and is even more necessary because of medicine's historical colonial posture. In recruiting participants, we were clear that we wanted to engage various voices, especially those that did not align with heteronormative frameworks. Thankfully, our storytellers heeded the call and came into community with us to share their experiences. We engaged everyone from those who were queer or gender nonbinary, to those who experienced or were experiencing mental and physical disabilities, addiction, HIV, or weight stigma, to those who had been incarcerated, and more. The bringing together of these individuals in community was inherently a decolonial act, and our time together was shaped by it. Rather than overly guide the group conversations, I and my co-researchers in the Livable Black Futures Storytelling Project let conversation flow where it needed to at the time. We were less invested in constructing linear stories legible to the mainstream. Instead we embraced the messiness of our lives and our histories. This was moving us toward the realization of the radical *we* necessary for reproductive justice work.

One thread that runs through the traumatic experiences that I encountered in both the stories of our storytellers and the stories I had read in articles and books was health care providers' intolerance for "messiness"—the complex bodies and contexts that patients brought into the medical space. Many described being met with frustration when their circumstances required more thought and creativity as opposed to standardized care. Eve Purdy calls for the appreciation of alternate ways of knowing in biomedicine and an embrace of the discomfort that comes with complex medical problems. She says, "There is a driving central tenet that the patients we care for, and the people with whom we work, are human" and that their care requires continually learning and becoming familiar with human complexity.[9] An intolerance for messiness exists all around us, but it is key to confront it if we are to undo the colonial legacies present in medicine and society at large.

EMBRACING INTERDEPENDENCE AND MESSINESS

> We are each other's harvest: / we are each other's business: / we are each other's magnitude and bond.
> —Gwendolyn Brooks

The refusal to expand our conversations about reproductive justice beyond normative frameworks has deadly consequences. The virtual erasure of trans, nonbinary, disabled, and plus-size individuals from this discourse implicitly sends the message that these groups of folks are disposable. For Black people in particular, the politics of anti-Black disposability is a constant that we must contend with. Its greatest manifestations are police violence and negligence, and mistreatment within the medical space. Treva Lindsey writes about the anti-Black politics of disposability, asserting that Black life is situated outside of any notion of legal protection and is overindexed as criminal.[10] She also notes that within health care, marginalized folks experience extreme forms of patient blame that focus on "unhealthy people" rather than "unhealthy and untenable systems, structures and institutions."[11] More concretely, these unhealthy and untenable spaces are infused with not only racism but also ableism, fatphobia, homophobia, misogynoir, and transmisogynoir, to name a few forms of structural devaluation.

The story of Dallas woman DeeDee Hall is a representative case of the deadly consequences of transmisogynoir in medicine.[12] Her death can be located at the intersections of medicine, carcerality, racism, and bias. DeeDee was a transwoman (MTF) experiencing a mental health crisis for which police and medics were called to the scene. Although she would not have been subject to gynecological and obstetric care, her care in the health care system is indicative of the bias infused in medicine and its deadly consequences. This also tracks with the treatment that transmen and nonbinary individuals experience and the disregard for their lives when they encounter medicine. These stories inform each other, and DeeDee Hall deserves to be included in this conversation.

On May 26, 2022, DeeDee Hall died en route to the hospital after being restrained by Dallas police. Her death occurred just as we were wrapping up the Dallas-based Livable Black Futures Storytelling Project, in which we had explored stories of medical harm, including harm to those who were queer and gender nonbinary. The urgency of these issues felt incredibly close to home. DeeDee was our sister too. She had been accosted by Dallas police after it was reported that she was causing a disturbance and potentially was under the influence of alcohol or drugs. After collapsing during questioning, she was placed in an ambulance, and a spit hood (fabric sack used to prevent spitting or biting) was pulled over her head. Body camera footage revealed officers and the medic making jokes at DeeDee's expense, misgendering her, and calling her "bud" and "sir" as well as disregarding her pleas to have the spit hood removed because she couldn't breathe.[13] At one point, DeeDee declared, "I'm dying, I'm dying," and then "I'm dead," which was met with no response from the medic or police. DeeDee's family shared that she had been diagnosed with bipolar disorder and schizophrenia, which further compounded the difficulties she faced as a Black trans disabled person. Under these circumstances, DeeDee stood little chance of being treated with dignity and respect. Instead she was treated as disposable and died as a result of this treatment. To add insult to injury, on May 11, 2023, nearly a year after the deadly encounter, a grand jury failed to indict the medic and the officers responsible for DeeDee's death. This decision is a reminder of the way Black folks, especially those who contend with the social stigmas of racism, ableism, homophobia, transmisogynoir, and more, continue to be disregarded in spaces where they are most vulnerable. Even health professionals like the medic who attended to DeeDee are not equipped to provide the care that DeeDee and others like her deserve. The story also represents the intertwining of medicine and policing.[14]

DeeDee Hall's case constellates the shared issues within sexual and reproductive health that are a result of colonial, heteronormative logics in medicine. It is also instructive in demonstrating the importance of organizing across difference. In her field-shifting essay "The Master's Tools Will Never Dismantle the Master's House," Audre Lorde explains, "Within the interdependence of mutual (nondominant) differences lies that security which enables us to descend into the chaos of knowledge and return with true visions of our future, along with the concomitant power to effect those changes which can bring that future into being. Difference is that raw and powerful connection from which our personal power is forged."[15] Here Lorde raises up the generative and power-building capacity of interconnection across difference. Rather than see difference as a site of contention or a space to jockey for dominance, we should see it as a path to build collective and personal power in the face of oppression.

Injustices like the one that DeeDee Hall experienced speak to the urgent need to decolonize sexual and reproductive health. Although DeeDee was biologically born male, she occupied a non-normative identity that subjected her to medical mistreatment. The disregard for her life also intersects with the experiences of Black queer birthing people, who often experience discrimination and neglect when they encounter gynecological and obstetric medicine. They often have to fight for the legitimacy of their identities and their specificity. This is especially true for nonbinary individuals.

Returning to Marshall Green, their 2011 film *It Gets Messy in Here* offers deep insight into how non-normative bodies are met with hostility in many contexts and how this can be most dangerous in a medical context. *It Gets Messy in Here* is a Black trans feminist film that examines the experiences of Black and Asian American transgender men and masculine-of-center queer women in public bathrooms. Using the politicization of public bathrooms as a launching point, the film is a larger opening to explore the perils of society's commitment to colonial logics of gender categorization. The co-collaborators who are interviewed in the project discuss the various implications of occupying a gender-fluid or gender-nonconforming body—the dangers of refusing societal categorization, the intersecting oppressions of inhabiting a racialized gender-nonbinary body, and the strategies of survival they must use so they can live safely as themselves. Unfortunately, the issues that the film explores remain relevant because of the ongoing legislative assault on queer and trans rights,[16] the banning of books with queer subject matter,[17] the continual policing of public bathrooms, and the removal of Pride displays in companies like Target due to disgruntled customers who have threatened employees.[18] This hostility is not exclusive to the aforementioned settings. In medical and birthing communities, queer and trans folk experience ongoing harm that often gets underreported, especially in relation to Black birthing outcomes.

In fact, if we shift the setting from the public bathroom to the examination table in a doctor's office, much of the content of *It Gets Messy in Here* still applies. Medical spaces are often sites of such heteronormativity—inherent in the separation of women's health and men's health. Trans folk often report experiences of discrimination, hostility, and even a refusal of health care due to their being gender nonconforming. Often, for a queer person, going to the gynecologist is a messy experience, and many elect to not seek health care because of the trauma they often experience in medical settings. These realities point to the multiple layers of erasure that trans folk experience in medicine. Whether because their identities are not acknowledged or because they are excluded from studies on sexual and reproductive health, queer and trans folk are rarely accounted for in conversations on maternal mortality and morbidity, much less Black queer and trans folk.

A 2022 study noted that lesbian and bisexual individuals were more likely to have children of low birth weight or stillborn.[19] And LGBTQ+ birthing people experience delays and denials in health care provision that can result in a slow death overall.[20] We know that life expectancy for LGBTQ+ folks is low. A 2014 study noted that living in communities hostile to LGBTQ+ individuals shortens their life span,[21] and across the board research studies on the Black birthing crisis acknowledge that LGBTQ+ individuals are underrepresented or even absent altogether from the data. In absence of representation in the data, poets like KB Brookins aim to bring greater awareness to these experiences for more inclusive conversations on sexual and reproductive health. Their poem "Sexting at the Gynecologist" is one example:

Sexting at the Gynecologist
KB Brookins

A camera is what makes it porn right? I google as everyone
    in the reception area wonders what husband is waiting for
    his wife.

Between my legs is a national treasure or at least what gives
republicans wet dreams during seasons of political theatre in
    Texas. Can I carry

that energy into a pose that reads digital exchange of chemistry?
    The tiny bathroom mirror says yes. My lover opens the text as
    some other kind of camera enters the canal that never wanted
    this. The same way republicans never want their donors to
    think they care about trans people. If I blur

the silhouette, is it still considered erotica? I think so,
said the nurse answering a separate question about my womb. If
    cameras

create the crime then I declare my pants untenable by white people
    unless they're doing routine checkups in a doctor's office. At
    least here,

the lobby thinks I'm offering moral support. And in a way, tea and
    a backrub
says everything okay just as much as my lover, eyes spangled
    when I show her what Dan Patrick hates.[22]

In spite of their marginalization in reproductive and sexual health settings and discourse, queer folk are speaking up about their experiences and making their experiences visible in the discourse. Brookins, a Texas-based, Black queer poet, writes powerfully about the stigma they experience going to the gynecologist. Although they are gender nonbinary, they go to the gynecologist for medical checkups in case they want to have children. They describe the process of trying to find a trans-friendly gynecologist and express that doing so is nearly impossible. Even after working to find a trans-friendly gynecologist, they experience misgendering there and questioning as to whether they belong. They're often called by their given name instead of their actual name. At the gynecologist, when asked "What are you needing today?," they reflect on possible answers: "I wish I could say understanding. I wish I could say someone I don't have to explain my humanity to. Someone with a more-than-101 understanding of what it means to be trans. Or what it means to be trans and Black and filled with fatigue. Someone wanting to be competent and humanlike to both demographics. Someone I trust to hug me."[23] KB highlights something key and unspoken in medicine—that it is an intimate and vulnerable experience. For medical practitioners it might just be another day at the office, but for patients this is often the first time in a while that they have been examined in their "private" areas. They lay themselves bare for strangers in the hopes of receiving care. When they receive the very opposite of that, it is traumatizing.

Storytellers in the Livable Black Futures Project reported similar experiences of feeling a lack of understanding and a general sense of un-belonging in gynecological and obstetric spaces. Queer individuals like Imani, a masculine-of-center woman, noted that they subconsciously avoid medical care, especially because being Black and queer makes it very difficult to find affirming medical care. Everything from the hostile looks they receive in the waiting room to the heteronormative questioning (assumptions about unplanned pregnancies and sexual activities) carries implicit messages that this is not a queer-friendly space. And in spite of this, queer storytellers know that it is important not to disengage from these spaces and that they deserve to be there like anyone else. Imani saliently noted that "even with the trauma of not being embraced in many medical spaces or many feminine spaces, [I still show] up because I still identify as a woman, I know I have needs, and still going and being there, and learning about my body, and being able to ask questions about my body that I couldn't really ask anybody else other than like reading through a biology textbook or something like that." Still showing up to receive support in exclusionary medical spaces signals a form of resistance and a refusal to be made invisible in sexual and reproductive health simply because one does not align with the heteronormative standard.

Increasingly, Black queer folks are making space for themselves in sexual and reproductive health work. In an interview entitled "Black-Led Queer and Trans Birth Work" for the podcast *Evidence Based Birth*, Black queer doulas Mystique Hargrove, Kortney Lapeyrolerie, and Nadine Ashby speak with Rebecca Dekker about what it is like to be Black queer birth workers when birth work remains focused on cisgendered women.[24] They speak about the isolation that comes with basic things such as the language that is used to talk about birth. Nadine Ashby notes that people feel threatened by inclusive language. The doulas discuss the multiple binds they face because of their positionality. They often experience racism in queer and trans communities and homophobia in Black communities. Because of this overwhelming feeling of exclusion and her desire to expand the conversation around birthing, Kortney Lapeyrolerie created the Queer Doula Network. She recalls in a doula training that she raised the point that trans folk have babies. The response to that was "Oh no, birth is a womanly experience." As a result of her refusal to align with that point of view, she was ostracized for the rest of the training. So she started the Queer Doula Network out of a sense of self-valuing and validating the experience of all birthing people. She says, "If nobody takes care of us and nobody heals us, we do that. We do that for each other." Here we see a move toward community care and self-care when dealing with a hostile world. This is the ethic that underscores reproductive justice—rather than work to fit within an exclusionary frame, these birth workers are creating spaces for themselves and in turn offering these kinds of transformative spaces for others.

CONFRONTING ABLEISM

Like the injurious and devastating outcomes of transphobia, homophobia, and heteronormativity in medicine more broadly, the convergence of various forms of systemic bias and ableism can have deadly effects when enacted in medical spaces. The 2020 emergency room death of Tashonna Ward, who had been diagnosed with an enlarged heart following a miscarriage, is one such example.[25] Ward had been experiencing debilitating effects from this condition but had received relatively little medical attention for the problem. She died after a two-hour wait in the ER, where she was never checked in and her case was never treated as an emergency. Black women are often perceived as medical "superbodies"[26] or as having little ability to feel pain. A study conducted by the Heller School for Social Policy and Management at Brandeis University found that Black disabled women have worse pregnancy outcomes than their white disabled peers, including higher medical expenses. Heidi Janz notes that medical ableism coupled with racism permeates the medical space and that these realities routinely make disabled people vulnerable in medical spaces.[27] In her analysis of Octavia Butler's *Fledging* and its depiction of the Black female disabled character Shori, Therí Pickens notes that the disabled Black female subject complicates the dialogue around race and disability. Notably, Pickens highlights the generative possibilities for deepening this discourse. She writes, "Racism and ableism vie for power over her [Shori's] body, and the places where they contradict each other and expose their instability. These contradictions open up space to imagine black female disabled subjects wielding radical political potential to build coalitions and alliances and to transform how others understand their positions in relation to privilege."[28] I am thinking again of the radical *we* that Marshall Green highlights and that animates this chapter. The storytelling of Black disabled birthing people creates even greater potential to organize across difference and to center the voices often marginalized in mainstream discourse.

Disability and sexuality educator Robin Wilson-Beattie offers a key illustrative example of the possibilities that open up when we complicate the discourse relating to Black sexual and reproductive health.[29] In a 2015 piece on her own abortion story, Wilson-Beattie brings to bear various vantage points all intersecting for her as a Black disabled queer polyamorous woman.[30] She conceived a child with someone other than her husband and decided to terminate the pregnancy. This decision was not made without deliberative thought. Already a mother to a three-year-old, Wilson-Beattie experienced complications from the spinal cord injury that had resulted in her disability, as well as preeclampsia and a post–cesarean section infection. Because of these issues, having a second child would present significant medical challenges that Wilson-Beattie didn't feel confident medical providers could handle in light of how they had handled her first pregnancy. In her search for options, she went to a traditional abortion clinic but was met with shame and stigma from the doctors. She was chided for getting pregnant given her spinal cord injury, and they refused to perform the abortion, saying it was too high risk and would need to be done in a hospital. She resented being told she shouldn't get pregnant because of her disability and rightly recognized the eugenic dimensions of such presumptions. Wilson-Beattie also reflects on the ways most medical providers actually encouraged her to get an abortion. She states: "People with disabilities are treated like we are not, a lot of times, by medical professionals or other people, like we are not complete people. Like we have something missing. When it comes to reproduction, we are encouraged not to. We are encouraged not to have children. We are encouraged not to reproduce." What Wilson-Beattie makes clear is that medical providers need to be equipped to handle the complex needs of disabled birthing people instead of discouraging them from reproduction because their bodies don't align with a heteronormative, ableist standard. Tien Sydnor-Campbell also offers insight into how little medical attention is paid to the Black woman's bodymind and the mental and physical care needs of Black birthing people navigating sexuality and disability.[31] She cites an overall inattentiveness to Black disabled birthing people, including a lack of effective guidance on accessible and safe sexual devices, positions, and access needs during pregnancy and delivery. The absence of education relating to these matters in medical spaces further adds to the stigma that Black disabled birthing people navigate.

Offering a historical context for the intersections of race, gender, and ableism in medicine, Mary Crossley notes the covert eugenic spirit in medicine that is felt very deeply by Black birthing people with disabilities, who already have histories of coercive sterilization. A notable case is the Relf sisters.[32] Minnie Lee and Mary Alice Relf, who were twelve and fourteen years old respectively when they were involuntarily sterilized by tubal ligation, became the poster children for the egregious practices of sterilization of Black girls and women during the 1960s and '70s. Both sisters had been labeled mentally disabled and targeted for sterilization by a federally funded family planning clinic in Montgomery, Alabama. Their case received national attention when the Relf family filed a class action lawsuit against Caspar Weinberger, the secretary of the Department of Health, Education and Welfare, and Alvin J. Arnett, then director of the Office of Economic Opportunity, for misuse of federal funds to enact harmful methods of birth control, including coerced sterilization. The *Relf v. Weinberger* (1973) case resulted in a prohibition against the use of federal funds for involuntary sterilization. Crossley makes the point that centering disability in reproductive justice discourse and advocacy can foster greater solidarity that "may produce progress toward specific policy and material goals" as well as enhance the dignity of those who often experience indignities in medical spaces.

Loretta Ross espouses similar sentiments as she notes disingenuous arguments that "abortion is racist" given the history of eugenics and efforts to suppress Black reproduction. Ross herself is a victim of such practices. She was involuntarily sterilized at the age of twenty-three.[33] Drawing on her personal experience and histories of Black women resisting eugenics, she reminds us that the "dual value system [the right to have a child or the right not to have a child] seeded an expanded vision of reproductive justice that guides the work of women of color today."[34] At the heart of this conversation is reproductive autonomy and the right to be seen as a whole person capable of making one's own decisions about one's life.

ADDRESSING HIV STIGMA

In addition to the intersections of ableism and queerphobia, the stigma of HIV contributes to the devaluation of Black birthing people and their relative exclusion from discourses about Black sexual and reproductive health. Seeking to address this disregard are individuals like Masonia Traylor and Ciara "Ci Ci" Colvin, who are both featured in the 2024 documentary *Unexpected*. Produced by Sheryl Lee Ralph and her nonprofit DIVA, the film follows the advocacy work of Traylor and Colvin, both of whom are Black mothers living with HIV. They met because they shared similar stories of being diagnosed with HIV during pregnancy. Together they provide support to mothers in rural Georgia through care packages and peer support in order to address the isolation and stigma that comes with living with HIV. Traylor laments the silencing surrounding HIV with respect to sexual and reproductive health. She says that although Black women are being infected at high rates, "Women are losing their lives and not sharing their stories." Here she speaks to the role of community voices in supporting one another. Through sharing their stories, Black women with HIV are able to help each other locate supportive providers and resources that can often mean the difference between life and death. Dazon Dixon Diallo, one of the speakers in the film, affirms that "who feels it knows it," so that it is important to look to Black women as partners in addressing ways to effectively care for people living with HIV. Dixon Diallo offers two key adages that affirm this approach: "When you service a woman, you service a community" and "If you fix it for Black women, you fix it for everyone." In all, the film *Unexpected* reminds us of the need to prioritize the voices of those experiencing the issues and treat them as experts to advance their own well-being.

Black birthing people make up two-thirds of diagnosed cases of HIV and only 13 percent of the US female population. Women aged twenty-five to sixty-four in this demographic are 8.2 times more likely to die of HIV than their white counterparts despite effective highly active antiretroviral therapy (HAART).[35] These realities place them at the heart of the Black maternal mortality crisis, yet they are often marginalized out of the conversation. In fact, the 2022 Texas Maternal Mortality and Morbidity Review Committee and Texas Department of State Health Services *Joint Biennial Report* noted that the maternal death rate in Texas is increasing, with 20.2 maternal deaths per 100,000 live births. Non-Hispanic Black women experienced the highest rates of severe maternal morbidity, with North Central Texas being one of the regions that had the highest rates.[36] These data, however, did not indicate if any of the individuals in the report were living with HIV. When these identities are not named and the data are overgeneralized, conversations about those who are multiply marginalized are limited.

The lack of concrete data on the role of HIV in the numbers driving the Black maternal mortality crisis only exacerbate the silences that still remain around HIV. The Livable Black Futures Storytelling storytellers who were living with HIV described alienation they experienced during and after pregnancy. Instead of encountering the attitude that birth was a joyful experience, they were often admonished to abort the baby, and if they did give birth, they were made to feel unworthy of being a mother. Research shows that because of various levels of structural oppression, Black birthing people living with HIV navigate issues of racism and discrimination that contribute to heightened stigmatization and make them more likely to experience depression, posttraumatic stress disorder, and substance abuse.[37]

Although we need more stories on the experiences of Black birthing people in the United States who are living with HIV, films such as June Cross's *Wilhemina's War* (2015) shines a light on this persistent issue from the perspective of those living in the US South, namely South Carolina.[38] Wilhemina Dixon herself is a grandmother caring for five people in her family who are living with HIV. The film explores the social isolation and stigma that come with being HIV positive. There are also issues of medical access and a lack of social supports such as transportation that makes it more difficult to access medical care. In the opener, Vivian Clark-Armstead of the South Carolina HIV/AIDS Council impresses upon the audience the urgency of addressing HIV. She makes the point that as with Black people abandoned during Katrina, no one is going to come and save them. The film also traces the feelings of abandonment after then governor Nikki Haley refused billions of dollars provided through the Affordable Care Act that would have given life-saving support to those dealing with issues of health access and economic inequality. This kind of neglect on the part of politicians more invested in political gamesmanship than in people further sends the message that people living with HIV are seen as disposable.

COMBATING WEIGHT STIGMA

An additional glaring but underengaged area of intersectional medical indignity is weight stigma. Weight stigma is a major area of medical indignity related to sexual and reproductive health. Nearly one in five birthing people have reported experiencing weight stigma in health care settings.[39] Researchers May Friedman, Carla Rice, and Emily Lind make the important point that "from a reproductive justice perspective, it is critical to note how anti-obesity discourses position certain populations as 'risk populations'—including women and transpeople . . . racialized and Indigenous peoples, and the working class/poor."[40] These foci reproduce stereotypes and target behaviors of these groups instead of the structural inequities they experience.

This subject is close to home for me here in Fort Worth, Texas, where maternal morbidity and mortality statistics are very high. Black birthing people in particular are imperiled by these realities. I remember reading an article written by two white women medical professionals in Fort Worth who cited obesity as a leading cause of Black maternal morbidity and mortality.[41] The article engaged in patient blame on levels that deeply disturbed me. Since that article, others have been written that take into account systemic racism and access to medical care; however, the conversation on medical bias and intersectional indignity experienced in medical spaces remains underdeveloped. Like those who experience homophobia, transphobia, and ableism in medicine, those who are plus-sized often avoid medical spaces because they are mistreated there. One disturbing aspect of the limited conversation on weight stigma as a reproductive justice issue is the lack of research on weight stigma as a contributing factor to poor outcomes for birthing people with higher-than-average BMI (Body Mass Index) numbers. What we do know is that there are connections between high BMI in birthing people and negative pregnancy outcomes. A 2021 study by Monica Saucedo et al. researching birthing people in France concluded that the risk of maternal death increases with BMI.[42] Correspondingly, US-based studies (such as the 2022 study by Frey et al) found that maternal prepregnancy obesity was associated with severe maternal morbidity and mortality.[43]

What often goes underdiscussed and underconsidered, however, is the role that weight stigma plays in the rates of poor maternal outcomes for plus-sized birthing people, especially Black plus-sized birthing people. This is an illustration of intersectional medical indignity and its dire consequences for Black birthing people. Exploring the experiences that Black plus-sized birthing people face unlocks key conversations and analyses that help us to undo much of the medical harm that we see. So many medical harm experiences converge on the Black body, and we need to center those who are multiply marginalized and Black. Blackness is a consistently marginalized identity in medicine, and we need to continue to draw attention to this.

The experience of being a fat, Black, disabled birthing person is expressed compellingly in the story of Dr. Angela Mack, one of the facilitators of the Livable Black Futures Project, who like many of us is personally implicated in this work. Mack is a scholar, poet, storyteller, and community educator. She generously shared with me the story of her personal involvement in the issues highlighted by the Livable Black Futures Project and what she hopes to see come from its efforts. We began by discussing her experience of learning she was pregnant. She described first being discouraged to reproduce—much as we see in the narratives of disabled birthing people. Angela described a "trajectory of doom" being laid out for her by the health professionals who treated her.

In her facilitation work, Angela served as a conduit for participants to tell what Friedman, Rice, and Lind describe as "reclamation stories"[44] in an attempt to heal from the harm they experienced from intersectional medical indignities. Angela brilliantly links these experiences to weight in her metaphor of "carrying weight." She says:

> Usually when someone who is seen or interpreted as obese or fat or plus size or curvy (the spectrum of language that comes with that), usually the way people understand weight is just by pounds.... But weight is not just material. There is often trauma connected to those pounds (racialized harm, social stigma, etc.). There's a history that's connected to those pounds. So when a person is carrying weight, you just see the physical. You don't see all they are carrying.

This reflects the concept of waterbreaking and all that is pent up within our bodies that we carry within us as a result of bearing these histories of medical harm. Angela also offers: "You know, sometimes a person, the weight that a person carries is whatever they've survived." Angela theorizes carrying weight as a host of confluences often met on the body. What she also reminds us is that we can't reduce individuals to stereotypes based on their size, and that we also have to affirm fatness as a body-positive framework that isn't necessarily bound up in trauma.

With this method and theory, Angela led our storytelling in a teardrop exercise that I can now only describe as a waterbreaking ceremony. Angela distributed symbolic tears cut out on pieces of construction paper. On one side, she had the participants write out whatever pain had been a part of their experience of being Black birthing people—to write out the story, mark it up, and release all the anger. Following that, we were to shed the tears by holding the paper over the trash can, releasing our stories silently or out loud, and then ripping up the paper. The room went quiet as storytellers wrote detailed thoughts on the pains they had experienced. I looked around and saw a beautiful collective of thinkers and healers working to shed the harm done by intersectional medical indignities and traumas (a radical *we*). We were queer, disabled, weight stigmatized, living with HIV, and more. Angela then invited us to share what we had written on our teardrops. Initially people were reluctant to share because saying out loud all of this pain has a risk of reopening the wound, and many of us had never healed from it or shared it out loud before. But eventually, in the safety of the room, we found the words to move us toward healing. One by one, each storyteller shared their pain, and one of our first speakers ended their story with a form of release that they couldn't fully find the words to express. In what was akin to the Black church call-and-response form of outcry, another storyteller in the room, Jade, proclaimed, "Fuck it." And the rest of us affirmed this. Our earlier storyteller affirmed it as well, saying, "Fuck it" as they ripped up their teardrop. We continued this way until everyone had finished. It was our flooding.

CHAPTER TWO

Reproductive Justice

An American Grammar

Affirmation
I take back my power through language, undoing binary logics that do not account for the fullness of who I am and my revolutionary capacity.

At a July 2022 Senate hearing about the impact of the Supreme Court's decision to reverse *Roe v. Wade*, scholar Khiara Bridges and Missouri senator Josh Hawley had a revealing exchange regarding perceptions about who can become pregnant. During the questioning, Hawley asked Bridges why she used the phrase "people with a capacity for pregnancy" when she discussed the impacts of abortion restrictions and bans.[1] Hawley was confused as to why Bridges would not simply say "women." Bridges explained that cisgendered women are not the only people capable of pregnancy: so are transmen and those who are nonbinary. When Hawley pushed back against Bridges's inclusive framing, she explained to him that his line of questioning was transphobic and "opens up trans people to violence." This exchange is emblematic of the power of language when it comes to matters of sexual and reproductive health. Khiara Bridges provided a master class for the world on the importance of naming for addressing oppression.

The issue of naming has been key to Black experience, especially for Black women, who have been marked by various stereotypes but whose subjectivities have not been truly accounted for. Hortense Spillers highlights this in her germinal essay "Mama's Baby, Papa's Maybe: An American Grammar Book." She opens the essay with the now oft-cited line: "Let's face it. I am a marked woman, but not everybody knows my name. 'Peaches' and 'Brown Sugar,' 'Sapphire' and 'Earth Mother,' 'Aunty,' 'Granny,' God's 'Holy Fool,' a 'Miss Ebony First,' or 'Black Woman at the Podium': I describe a locus of confounded identities, a meeting ground of investments and privations in the national treasury of rhetorical wealth."[2] This litany of names represents all the ways naming has been used to contain and limit Black women's voices and agency. Even when originally inscribed as terms of endearment, the labels become collapsed into flattened caricatures of Black womanhood that also alienate Black women from the category of woman. Spillers calls the writing of her essay an effort to produce an "American grammar" that is really a "rupture and a radically different kind of cultural continuation."[3] It is an attempt to express the fact that we have to make room in our language for the different kind of female subject that emerges from the transatlantic slave trade and into the present. Doing so enables a figure like "Sapphire" to write "a radically different text for female empowerment."[4] When we consider how language can provide a full account of the experiences of Black birthing people in mainstream discourse, it is clear that new words have to be invented and new names have to be used to fully empower subjects marginalized within white patriarchal and heteronormative frameworks.

Christina Sharpe offers the term *anagrammatical blackness* to describe the way that language needs to be reoriented to fully articulate blackness and Black relationality. Following the line of Spillers, and noting how gender gets disrupted during transatlantic slavery alongside familial relations, particularly the relation of mother and child, Sharpe explains that in this context, "grammatical gender falls away and new meanings proliferate."[5] She asks a key question: "What new words do we need?"[6] Also, how must we think relations that can be potentially invaded by property relations? To this extent, by invoking a grammar of reproductive justice, I am thinking of it as an anagrammatical lexicon that disrupts language used to manage, confine, and control marginalized folks, particularly Black people. It is an "index of violability and also potentiality," as Sharpe would have it.[7] This chapter catalogs the terms that marginalized Black birthing people use to name themselves and their conditions, as well as key terms used in relation to reproductive justice. In doing so, the chapter gathers key terms for the conversations informing this book and broader discussions about reproductive justice. While not fully comprehensive, it maps out the key ideas animating this work. It is my goal that this grammar will become a tool for teaching and thinking reproductive justice.

IDENTIFIERS

WOMBHOLDER This word was invented out of the desire (within the Livable Black Futures Storytelling Project and in various spaces working toward sexual and reproductive liberation) to use a term that would account for all those implicated in conversations on sexual and reproductive health—not just those who identified as cisgendered women. Melissa Muganzo-Murphy, executive producer of the film *The Big Hysto: A Black Womb Revolution*, uses this term in the film. It has grown in usage across various platforms and has resonated in our community deeply.

BIRTHING PEOPLE This is a gender-inclusive term to name those who give birth regardless of their gender identification. I use it throughout the book as a way to consistently reference the individuals I engage with in the work. Like *wombholder*, this term is nascent in its usage but is gaining traction in the public sphere. Yet terms like these get significant pushback. In 2021, Congresswoman Cori Bush received backlash on social media about her use of the term.[8] Most recently, scholar Khiara Bridges sparred with Senator Josh Hawley, who challenged her use of gender-inclusive language such as *people with the capacity for pregnancy*, as mentioned above. Other terms include *uterus-bearing individuals* and *pregnant people*.[9]

GENDERQUEER, NONBINARY Although many definitions abound for these terms, *genderqueer* and *nonbinary* primarily refer to those whose gender identity doesn't fully align with the concept of man or woman. Marshall Green's film *It Gets Messy In Here* is a comprehensive resource for terms such as these. The film brings forward other terms such as *stud, boi, gender-fluid*, and *masculine of center* to demonstrate the resistance to definitions and labels as a rejection of heteronormative logics.

WEIGHT STIGMATIZED This book uses the term *weight stigmatized* to name the harmful treatment of those who identify as *fat, plus-sized,* and *bigger-bodied*. I use this term when discussing weight stigma in medicine; however, I affirm the claiming of terms such as *fat* that have been historically meant to cause emotional harm.[10]

BLACK GYNECOLOGICAL PUBLICS A diverse collective of voices speaking (or articulating) a Black feminist ethic of reproductive justice that is fully inclusive and invested in advancing an anticolonial approach to medicine that addresses historical and ongoing harm.

STORYTELLING

WATERBREAKING I coin this term in the introduction of this book as a way to describe the generative process that comes from breaking the silence about Black experiences with sexual and reproductive health. Drawing on the many valences of water primarily in the birthing experience and in Black culture, from the Middle Passage to Hurricane Katrina, Flint, Michigan, Jackson, Mississippi, and beyond, I consider how water has been central to shaping Black movement and social movements. Invoking water as a metaphor in this way ties together the collective force of Black storytelling and the birthing of change out of the waters of social movements such as reproductive justice.

AFTERMEMORY I conceive of this idea as a play on both Morrison's concept of "rememory" and "afterbirth" (the expelling of the placenta after the baby has been delivered). "Aftermemory" is the residue of releasing painful memories—those inside you that you have to nurse individually through the placenta of your inner life. When we release those memories into the world, we hold them up to others for them to also see and reckon with. We no longer need to provide them with just our oxygen—bearing them in our silence. When we tell our stories with intention and to those who desire to preserve them, we are engaging in aftermemory work. I discuss this in greater depth in chapter 3.

CRITICAL FABULATION Saidiya Hartman coined this term as a way to describe her process of storytelling in her engagement with the transatlantic slavery archive. She writes,

By playing with and rearranging the basic elements of the story, by re-presenting the sequence of events in divergent stories and from contested points of view, I have attempted to jeopardize the status of the event, to displace the received or authorized account, and to imagine what might have happened or might have been said or might have been done. By throwing into crisis "what happened when" and by exploiting the "transparency of sources" as fictions of history, I wanted to make visible the production of disposable lives (in the Atlantic slave trade and, as well, in the discipline of history), to describe "the resistance of the object," if only by first imagining it, and to listen for the mutters and oaths and cries of the commodity.[11]

I draw on Hartman's strategy to consider the archive of medical records where the voices of Black patients are often obscured in favor of the accounts of the authors, who are medical practitioners. I think on how storytelling serves as a way to enact resistance to archival silence, though the stories may differ from what enslaved subjects experienced.

COLLECTIVE REMEMORY In chapter 3, I conceive of collective rememory as the constancy of Black experience that cannot be lost despite efforts to suppress it. Encounters with these sites of memory prompt a communal reckoning with the past. Riffing off Toni Morrison's notion of rememory, I expand this concept beyond the singular to think about the impact of the resonance of memory in landscapes and in various sites.

ENDARKENED STORYWORK Thinking with scholars such as Cynthia B. Dillard and her path-making research on endarkened feminist epistemology in qualitative research and communal practices like Indigenous storywork, S.R. Toliver defines endarkened storywork as an approach to research that "requires that we listen to our research partners, ourselves, and our world, considering the connections between the story, storyteller, story listener, cultural traditions, and spiritual relationships in a field that asks us to view people as bounded, autonomous individuals."[12]

IMAGINATION In recent discourse, imagination has been a key part of the critical work of Black storytelling. Thinker and activist adrienne maree brown explains, "We are in an imagination battle. Trayvon Martin and Mike Brown and Renisha McBride and so many others are dead because, in some white imagination, they were dangerous."[13] The political dimensions of imagining have been espoused by scholars such as Robin D.G. Kelley and his notion of "freedom dreams," Lucille Clifton, Octavia Butler, Toni Morrison, Ruha Benjamin, and Mariame Kaba, to name a few. See also chapter 4, "Imagining Livable Black Futures," for further elaboration on this concept.

BODILY AUTONOMY

REPRODUCTIVE OPPRESSION (AND COERCION) Loretta Ross and Rickie Solinger explain, "The American Congress of Obstetricians and Gynecologists has declared that 'controlling the outcomes of a pregnancy, coerc[ing] a partner to have unprotected sex and interfer[ing] with contraceptive methods' all constitute reproductive coercion."[14] They say that the development of various assisted reproductive technologies and other innovations poses medical, ethical, and capitalist concerns regarding who is implicated in the right to be a mother or parent. In this sense, the various forms of coercion can be carried out in the interests of the state (or by the state). This is also a form of what Ross and Solinger call reproductive management and pregnancy policing.

REPRODUCTIVE AUTONOMY This wide-ranging term has been theorized in many spaces, but I rely chiefly on Dorothy Roberts's work tracing the history of the way Black reproduction has been subject to government repression and interference. She extensively explores this in *Killing the Black Body*, where she details the impact of the use of harmful contraceptives like Norplant and Depo Provera as well as the degradation and criminalization of Black motherhood. Roberts also explores threats to reproductive autonomy in her book *Torn Apart: How the Child Welfare System Destroys Black Families—and How Abolition Can Build a Safer World*. By interrogating the child welfare system, we see an extension of the state into the lives of Black families, intervening in their reproductive liberty. These issues are also especially urgent given the attempts to legislate against gender-affirming care and other forms of bodily autonomy.

CARE

BLACK TRANS FEMINISM I rely on Marquis Bey's theorization in their book *Black Trans Feminism* as an unfixing of blackness, gender, and feminism from static categories. It is an intervention in feminism as an ideological project and pushes against those borders as a project of abolition and gender radicality. A response to trans antagonism and exclusions of trans folk from feminist organizing, Black trans feminism constitutes radical freedom.[15]

RADICAL WE Although the concept of the radical *we* has been defined in other conversations on organizing across difference, particularly Audre Lorde's theory of interdependence, Kai Marshal Green informs my usage of the term as an articulation of solidarity. They write: "The Black feminist call for an androgynous self is a call to recognize the *them/we* always present in the I which seemed to be forgotten when all the *women* were thought to be white and all the Blacks were thought to be men in social and political thought and praxis."[16] Black feminist interruptions in these rigid categories open space for a radical *we* to emerge.

BIRTH JUSTICE My use of this term is informed by the movement to decolonize birth led by organizations such as Voices for Birth Justice, the Southern Roots Doula Collective, Black Women's Birth Justice, SisterSong, and individuals such as Ericka Hart (mentioned earlier) who advocate for full inclusion in birth work regardless of gender or sexuality. Voices for Birth Justice offers a concise definition of this term: "To challenge systems of oppression, such as racism and sexism in reproductive care, Birth Justice advocates for culturally-appropriate, person-centered care while challenging disrespectful care. It also supports the sharing of knowledge amongst communities and improves access to breastfeeding support and traditional birth-workers, such as midwives and doulas."[17] This includes validation of ancestral knowledges and anticolonial methods of enacting care.

HEALING JUSTICE Healing justice is a concept formed and explained by Cara Page and Erica Woodland in their collection *Healing Justice Lineages: Dreaming at the Crossroads of Liberation, Collective Care, and Safety*. In summary, they define it as a community-led response to intervene on individual and collective trauma; an emergent process to address various forms of historical and current trauma; a spiritual framework that seeks to remember the ancestral traditions of survival; a cultural strategy that seeks to create models of holistic care and safety; a political strategy to decriminalize communal care practices and ancestral traditions; and a challenge to the medical-industrial complex and the pervasiveness of bias against multiply marginalized individuals.

SOCIAL AND STRUCTURAL DETERMINANTS OF HEALTH Researchers Joia Crear-Perry et al. write in their piece "Social and Structural Determinants of Health Inequities in Maternal

Health" that we have to think beyond the social determinants of health often invoked in institutions as the basic needs for human thriving. These are incomplete because individuals are unlikely to be able to control directly many of the upstream determinants of health: governance, policy, and cultural or societal norms and values that shape who has access to health-promoting resources and opportunities and who does not. Beginning from this vantage point allows an understanding of why social determinants are born from structural determinants and cannot be addressed separately. In other words, no matter how empowered, knowledgeable, or willing someone is to change their behavior, they may not be able to do so because of structural determinants of health inequities.[18]

STIGMA AND BIAS

MEDICAL ABLEISM Heidi L. Janz notes that "health care professionals tend to underestimate substantially the quality of life of people with disabilities,"[19] although they often shape the way decision-makers, legislators, families, and society in general think about and sense disability. This has tremendous consequences, including negative health outcomes due to the stigma of disability that permeates medicine. I explore additional theorizations of this term and draw on Tien Sydnor-Campbell's illuminating discussion of the underlying issues for Black-identified women seeking support for sexual and reproductive health. She states:

> Knowing that there are relatively no examples of disabled beauty in print/electronic media, culture, or educational settings leaves a large population without representation. The DBW [disabled Black woman] is one of the least represented groups in western culture. The disabled Black woman, who does not speak up or out, is not

seen as having sex or sexuality issues. Additionally, these women are not even typically treated for sex or sexuality issues; socially, mentally/emotionally, or physically. The caveat being different unless obstetrics is concerned.[20]

This is a dimension of medical ableism that has particularly dire consequences for disabled Black birthing people.

WEIGHT STIGMA May Friedman et al. make the point that "weight bias—embedded into health care spaces (small chairs and inaccessible tables and tools in doctors' offices); technologies (ultrasound equipment that does not fit fat bodies; technologists unskilled in manual palpation of fat flesh), and provider policies, attitudes and practices—multiplies and magnifies with each occurrence."[21] This produces shame and stress and ultimately blocks access to care.

INTERSECTIONAL MEDICAL INDIGNITY I developed this term to name the way various biases in medicine can often converge on one body and cause harm to the individual (for instance, if one is Black, disabled, and queer). Too often, conversations about these forms of bias treat them as separate issues. Extending the issues Kimberlé Crenshaw and other Black feminists aimed to raise in their creation of terms such as *intersectionality* and *the double bind*, the concept of intersectional medical indignity is an attempt to account for the experiences in medicine of multiply marginalized individuals with greater depth than we do currently. Not doing so often results in "intersectional invisibility"—the virtual absence of those who inhabit multiply marginalized identities from conversations about medicine or in the research.

CARCERALITY

MEDICAL-INDUSTRIAL COMPLEX Cara Page, in *Healing Justice Lineages*, makes the point that we have to situate medicine within conversations about profits and policing that have "impacted our communities for centuries as an extension of state control, capitalism, and exploitation through racist/ableist science."[22] This system relies on heteronormative notions of health and illness; prescribes who is expendable; determines whose bodies are criminalized and pathologized; functions as an extension of state control and violence; and criminalizes traditions outside the practice of Western medicine.

AFTERLIVES OF SLAVERY Saidiya Hartman provides this key term for describing the ongoing effects of transatlantic slavery on the descendants of those who were enslaved. She makes the point that Black life is still imperiled by a political arithmetic entrenched centuries ago. She writes, "This is the afterlife of slavery—skewed life chances, limited access to health and education, premature death, incarceration and impoverishment."[23]

ABOLITION MEDICINE Abolition medicine is an effort to render visible how carceral logics operate in medicine and uses the methodology of abolition to undo those logics. Yoshiko Iwai, Zahra H Khan, and Sayantani DasGupta explain:

> The essential work of abolition medicine is to interrogate the upstream structures that enable downstream violence, like police brutality, in addition to reimagining the work of medicine altogether as an anti-racist practice. Abolition medicine means challenging race-based diagnostic tools and treatment guidelines that reinforce antiquated and scientifically inaccurate notions of biological race. It means integrating longitudinal anti-racist training into medical education, including the history of racism in medicine and structural factors that produce racial health disparities, while actively recruiting, retaining, and supporting Black and other minoritised faculty, staff, and students. Supporting institutional efforts that provide reparations to communities of colour devastated by unethical medical experimentation, such as the class action lawsuit that ultimately awarded monetary restitution and a lifetime of free medical care to the families involved in the

Tuskegee Study, is another instrument of social change for abolition medicine, as is advocating for universal health coverage. And these changes are only a beginning. Importantly for us, practising abolition medicine entails health workers joining national conversations about police abolition and using their social power to reinvest in programmes that build community capacity for mental health care, youth development, education, and employment, as well as harm reduction efforts around drug use, housing insecurity, and incarceration.[24]

I quote this at length because this comprehensive definition speaks to the various issues that I raise in chapter 5 on carcerality.

CHAPTER THREE

Rememory

A Reproductive Justice Mixtape

Affirmation
I embrace myself unapologetically and release shame. Doing so honors the ancestors whose bodies and minds have been exploited for the development of gynecological medicine and who have endured histories of judgment and silencing.

The first thing we did was make a playlist. In preparation for the Livable Black Futures storytelling circles, we knew we needed music to guide the experience—music to write to, to cry to, to dance to, to release, to fill the silence. We included over one hundred songs, from Mary J. Blige's "My Life" to Tank and the Banga's "Dope Girl Magic" and Jhené Aiko's "Trigger Protection Mantra." Qiana took the lead in crafting a playlist that would be full of care and uplift. We also made space for what some might call revolutionary ratchetness,[1] an unapologetic space that was shame free and rooted in self-love. The silence-breaking impact of music cannot be overestimated. So much of the silence our storytellers experienced came from prior instances of being shamed and ashamed of their bodies and themselves. Moving through a society that was built on expectations of normativity and that always already treated sex and sexuality as shameful had a cumulative effect of making it difficult to speak freely about experiences with respect to sexual and reproductive health. Music was an entry point for our storytellers to gain insight into our methodological approach to this work. Although our method was organically formed, we were cultivating and enacting it through music.

Care was our starting point for establishing our method. We knew our key question: In naming our experiences of gynecological and obstetric violence, as well as institutional and medical racism, how can we imagine new possibilities of being and care that enable Black futures?

The next step for us would be to think about how we would get there. Because we were unearthing memories of harm, care was essential to supporting individuals who likely would experience triggers from revisiting these experiences. Moreover, since care had often been absent from these prior experiences, we wanted to use this space to practice what intentional care looked like.

Care served as a portal to offer a sense of safety and the creation of a space that allowed for the releasing of shame and stigma. Beyond care, we drew on other principles informed by our values to establish a space of safety. We approached this work from a communal perspective where we served as participant-researchers alongside those we welcomed in. We refused a hierarchical structure of knowledge production where the researchers served as the authority figures and primary interlocutors. Though we were always conscious of the researcher/participant dynamic, we did our best to establish values of shared expertise and the understanding that we all brought a certain degree of knowledge into the space. In producing a communal space, we were able to affirm our collective dignity and power as well as embodied knowledges. Importantly, we made the space as inclusive as possible with respect to sexuality, access to resources, and other factors that often limit research participants from engagement. Prioritizing inclusivity created a space where people who were genderqueer and nonbinary, lesbian, formerly incarcerated, living with HIV, underresourced, and more would feel supported and heard. A central point of pride from this work was that we were able to form a supportive and inclusive space where Black wombholders could feel empowered to speak about all the ways they had experienced harm in terms of their sexual and reproductive health.

So our playlist was a dynamic reflection of these values, and the music supported a communication of them in ways that reminded us about the power of creativity as a form of expressing the ineffable, as a facilitator of healing, as resistance, and as a cultural intervention, as Monica Simpson of SisterSong would have it.[2] Some lyrics, like those of Mary J. Blige's "My Life,"[3] supported internal reflection and were a prelude for storytelling. Other lyrics, like those of Tank and the Bangas's "Dope Girl Magic," took us to a place of confident expression and abundance.[4] That feeling of empowerment provided us with the strength to not only reflect on hard pasts but celebrate how far we had come from those pasts. And when the conversations became too much or too heavy, we used songs like Jhené Aiko's "Trigger Protection Mantra" to help us breathe. The repetition of the soothing lyrics was cleansing to our spirits.[5] Their assurance of protection stands in contrast to Malcolm X's proclamation that "the most unprotected person in America is the Black woman." And we know that both things can be true at the same time—that the United States is a site of harm for Black women but that we can find protection within ourselves and in one another. One storyteller even noted that music was a key part of her "trigger action plan," signaling the critical role of the sonic in healing. Music translated the ethos we wanted to create in the space. And in many ways the songs became reminders for us about what we were hoping to gain out of the journey and how we wanted to do our work.

This chapter details the ways various forms of Black feminist creativity (from music to visual art and literature) served, and continue to serve, as an anchor for our storytelling work. Engaging with this creative work facilitated expressive freedom, safety, and imagination for our storytellers. The waterbreaking that occurred in our meetings would not have been possible without Black feminist creativity, which often expressed the ineffable and gave language to the feelings our storytellers were endeavoring to communicate. In addition to exploring the liberating force of Black feminist creativity and its capacity to inspire informal storytelling work, this chapter examines the significance of formal storytelling practices on their own as a creative intervention into the challenges facing Black birthing people. In many respects, they serve as a creative form of sexual and reproductive liberation—of otherwise imagining, a life-giving force. I envision this chapter being read like a mixtape—an exploration of various forms of creative work in the service of bodily liberation and justice.

COLLECTIVE REMEMORY—A REMIX

Across my own exploration of the transformative force of Black creativity for reproductive justice, I have contemplated how creativity and memory can be and often are interconnected, especially with regard to the Black past, where archival record-keeping is limited and the imagination becomes one of the only ways to access ancestral experience. This was the challenge facing Toni Morrison when she wrote about her act of literary archaeology in going to the "site of memory" to imagine what the relics of the past were saying to her. It is also a part of her work in *Beloved*, where Sethe ruminates to her daughter Denver on the notion of "rememory": "Some things go. Pass on. Some things just stay. I used to think it was my rememory. You know. Some things you forget. Other things you never do. But it's not. Places, places are still there. If a house burns down, it's gone, but the place—the picture of it—stays, and not just in my rememory, but out there, in the world."[6] Denver asks Sethe if other people can see her rememory and Sethe responds, yes. She goes on to say that you can encounter other people's rememory because "even though it's all over—over and done with—it's going to always be there waiting for you."[7] This conversation signals how expansive the notion of rememory is and the various forms it can take. Morrison highlights the complexity of memory, whether it is memories of trauma that emerge at unexpected times or the layers of shared experience that live in the body politic and beyond the self, especially across generations. In line with Morrison's thought, Edwidge Danticat, in her work *Breath, Eyes, Memory*, shows the impact of transgenerational memory on the descendants of those who experienced trauma through her characters Sophie and Martine.[8] *Breath, Eyes, Memory* takes up the story of Sophie Caco, a Haitian immigrant to the United States whose life is shaped by her mother's rape by a member of the Haitian militia, the Ton Ton Macoutes, of which Sophie is a product. The trauma her mother experienced is inscribed on Sophie's life, and she must do her own healing work to recover. Writers like Morrison and Danticat grounded me in how I approached the relationship between memory, creativity, and storytelling for reproductive justice.

Artistic explorations of transgenerational and collective memory work were at the forefront of my mind when I witnessed the power of creativity, memory, and healing in Montgomery, Alabama, during the 2022 Anarcha Lucy Betsey Day of Reckoning Conference. The conference, an annual three-day summit centered on the history of American gynecology, provides, in the words of organizer and visionary Michelle Browder, "an opportunity for obstetricians, gynecologists, doulas, midwives, and medical practitioners to learn how to change the narrative in race in healthcare disparities."[9] I found this description to be true as I witnessed a powerful collectivity of researchers, health care providers, invested community members, and more. We had traveled far and wide—internationally and domestically—to be a part of this event. As we looked at the sea of people assembled, it was undeniable that Michelle Browder had done something transformative. It is rare to see this kind of diverse group (activists, medical practitioners, reproductive justice advocates, and more) working alongside one another and investing in Black birthing people's health and reproductive justice together. This year was particularly special because it was the inaugural event. Browder created an immersive experience of music, seminars, public lectures, and experiential engagements (including the official opening of the Mothers of Gynecology Park in the heart of Montgomery and a visit to the J. Marion Sims clinic where Sims had performed his experiments).

Michelle Browder's creative intervention serves as a foundation for the diverse and ongoing reckoning with harmful histories that still affect Black birthing people today. Browder ties creative arts to the work of changing the narrative, which is key because the central work of Black storytelling is that of changing the narrative. She characterizes her work as that of a "creative extremist," a term she takes from Martin Luther King's "Letter from a Birmingham Jail": "What the South need[s] more of are creative extremists. That let me know that I was OK to use my art to radically change the minds of people, and how they see people in this country and how they deal with them."[10] On her own, Michelle Browder is a transformative figure. She is a descendant of civil rights activists, including her father, Curtis Browder, the first Black person to serve as prison chaplain in the state of Alabama. Additionally, her aunt is Aurelia Browder, who was arrested for sitting in the white section of a city bus and was the plaintiff in *Browder v. Gayle*, the 1956 Alabama District Court case that ruled bus segregation unconstitutional, though it was swiftly undermined and successfully appealed by the state and upheld by the Supreme Court in the same year.[11] Against this backdrop Browder seeks to educate the public about critical histories and create art from it. Her company, "More Than Tours," takes visitors on a dynamic tour of key civil rights and Black historical landmarks across Montgomery. One can easily spot Browder's imprint by sculptural replicas of her signature red glasses that are placed around the city and in the iconography of More than Tours. Her red glasses signify a way of visualizing history through her lens[12] and giving viewers the chance to experience these historical moments through her eyes.

For many reasons, Michelle Browder's monument *Mothers of Gynecology* is an illuminating example of transgenerational memory work, or what we might think of as *collective rememory*. I conceive of collective rememory as the constancy of Black experience that cannot be lost to efforts to suppress it. Encounters with these sites of memory prompt a communal reckoning with the past. First, the monument sits in the heart of Montgomery, just a few miles from the clinic where J. Marion Sims conducted his experiments on enslaved women. Described by Browder as a "living memorial," the monument depicts Anarcha, Lucy, and Betsey, three named women who experienced Sims's brutal operations. The sculptures are a mixture of discarded items such as steel, surgical scissors, silk sutures, and bicycle chains (found in junkyards and through donation), welded together. Browder uses these materials to reconstruct the bodies of these women into visual images of empowerment, a form of these women gaining control over the instruments of their oppression. For instance, Browder made a tiara for Betsey out of a speculum—a medical tool that Sims is credited for inventing.

The visuals of the statues are multilayered.[13] These figures are imposing and vulnerable at the same time. Anarcha, the tallest statue, stands at fifteen feet (with Betsey and Lucy at twelve and nine feet, respectively). Anarcha holds her head proudly in the air, adorned with earrings that bear the Adinkra symbol *gye nyame*, meaning "But God"—an idea that surely resonates in a site like Alabama, where religion plays a key role in the culture. Incorporating the African imagery also ties the women to identities beyond enslavement. Additionally, there is a hole in the middle of Anarcha's statue, symbolizing a missing womb. The representative womb sits nearby on the ground, full of cut glass, needles, and other objects that represent the invasive and extensive medical experimentation on her body. Anarcha notably had the most surgeries (at least thirty).[14] These never resulted in a cure for vaginal fistulas, and she had to seek additional medical treatment.[15] Hair is also critical in the visual presentation of these historical figures. Anarcha's hair is in angular braids, Betsey's is in cornrows, and Lucy's is in Bantu knots. These styles, specific to Black culture, gesture to the

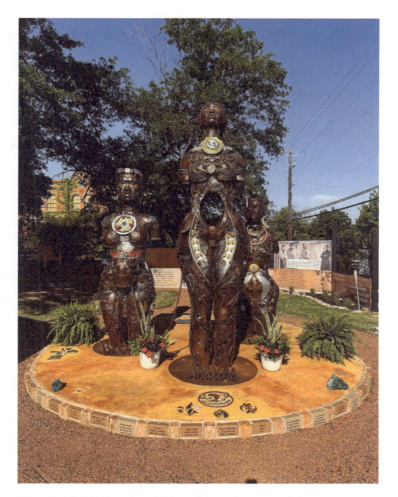

Figure 1. Michelle Browder's *Mothers of Gynecology* statues in Montgomery, Alabama. Artwork by Michelle Browder. Photo by Steven Zucker.

personhood of these women. They exude a regality that belies what their bodies have been through. In this way, Browder shifts the lens through which we see these three figures. This is critical work because Alabama remains a site of medical and racial inequality. Browder's work provides a new lens through which to see history and makes space for the possibility of contemporary repair.

Alongside the visuals, the statues have a textual quality. Ntozake Shange's words from *for colored girls who have considered suicide when the rainbow is enuf* supply the key messaging for the *Mothers* statues: "let her be born / let her be born and handled warmly."[16] These words imply care and support, which announces an intentionality in how visitors should engage with these statues and by extension Black birthing people being born in and giving birth under precarious conditions. On the site, Browder incorporates a space to contemplate and process the history one learns while at the statues, so it is also an act of care for those visiting. Names of various Black women are welded onto the statue, including names of Black writers, such as Sonia Sanchez; those who have lost their life in childbirth, such as Kira Johnson;[17] those who have endured difficult birth experiences, such as Serena Williams; and those who have been victims of police brutality and other forms of socially sanctioned violence against Black women, such as Sandra Bland. The collective of names provides another narrative dimension for this visual encounter.

The site-specific creative and cultural intervention of *Mothers of Gynecology* recognizes Montgomery as a location of an infamous history of medical harm against Black people. To return to Morrison's concept of "rememory"—the sense that places (like buildings and homes) can linger even if they are no longer standing and that even when we think something is "over and done with," it still remains waiting for us—this is what I am thinking of as I walk the streets of Montgomery. It is important to note that Montgomery is approximately a forty miles' drive from Tuskegee, the site of the infamous Tuskegee "Study of Untreated Syphilis in the Negro Male" conducted between 1932 and 1972 by the US

Public Health Service and the Centers for Disease Control and Prevention.[18] In this study, nearly four hundred Black research subjects were denied informed consent and were not offered treatment for syphilis even after it became available. Just after the study's closing year in Montgomery, Minnie Lee and Mary Alice Relf were sterilized without their consent in 1973 (as referenced in chapter 1 of this book). Walking around Montgomery, I could feel the weight of these histories. All around, one can see efforts to call attention to the historical harms embedded in the city's landscape.

The 2022 Anarcha Lucy Betsey Day of Reckoning Conference illuminated for me what it means to engage histories of medical exploitation in tangible ways and to utilize these painful encounters as catalysts to enact change. Deirdre Cooper Owens, one of the conference's keynote speakers, made this clear in her address. She talked about the challenges she faced getting support for her research on the ways Black enslaved women and Irish women were used and exploited for medical experimentation. Her book *Medical Bondage* explores these histories in ways that have transformed the discourse and field of medical historicizing. It is due to Cooper Owens's research and the work of scholars like Harriet Washington, whose book *Medical Apartheid* takes up histories of medical exploitation on Black Americans, that we have reached a cultural recognition and awareness of these histories and how they inform the delivery of modern medicine, particularly the way Black people experience medicine. During her speech, Cooper Owens made plain that it is not enough just to research and be aware of these histories: we have to think about what is owed to the victims of these brutal experiments and to their descendants. Cooper Owens's invitation to the audience to contemplate what it would mean to repair this damage, to redress this history, stuck with me not only because it was a powerful question but because it was one that felt overwhelming to answer. How do you repair this damage?

Almost as if anticipating Cooper Owens's words (a kind of Black feminist call and response), Browder offered her own intervention. During the conference, we learned that Browder had been able to secure purchase of Sims's clinic and planned to transform it into a medical healing space. In fact, following the conference, Browder announced the opening of the Mothers of Gynecology Health and Wellness Museum and Clinic to the public.[19] It will be a space to address medical apartheid in places like Alabama and will serve as a space for gynecologists, doulas, midwives, and various medical practitioners to offer primary and prenatal care to uninsured birthing people. It is also meant to be a space of education, healing, and hope. Not only is Browder performing this critical work, but she also held a Go Fund Me campaign for Minnie Lee and Mary Alice Relf that made it possible for the two sisters to purchase a house.[20] (Notably, in spite of the legal advocacy done on their behalf, the Relf sisters never received financial compensation for being sterilized by coercion.)

HOW CAN YOU MEASURE THIS PAIN?

Michelle Browder's commendable efforts provide a model for other forms of repair and invite the question: What does a broader institutional and national reckoning look like? What does it mean for medical institutions and the US government to truly be held accountable for and work to repair these past harms and their ongoing ripples? Bettina Judd's poetry collection *patient* meditates on this question through a form of creative rememory (or what she calls "after memory")—a reminder to us that if we don't remember this past, it will be co-opted and the narrative changed to one that further silences and obscures the voices of the past. *patient* is a project of recovery to tell the stories of victims of medical exploitation (namely Anarcha, Lucy, and Betsey—Sims's "patients"—as well as Joice Heth, Saartjie Baartman, and Henrietta Lacks).

Across the numerous poems exploring these figures and their legacies, there is a continual meditation on just how to measure pain. In "How to Measure Pain I" Judd writes:

> In the woman it is a checklist:
>
> Can you imagine anything
> worse than this?
>
> If the answer is no, ask again[21]

Judd's words speak to conversations about repair from historical injustices (whether slavery, Jim Crow, or the medical harms against Black people across time). Measuring just what damage has occurred is an overwhelming task. The query "Can you imagine anything / worse than this?" highlights the extent to which the pain Judd explores in the collection is unfathomable. We can infer that the unspoken answer to this query is "no" because Judd returns to this question later in the text in "How to Measure Pain II: Maggot Brain." The poem begins:

> "How do you   daughter measure pain?"[22]

This time, the question is posed to a "daughter" in a signal of transgenerational rememory but also a gesture to the legacy of such pain—recognizing that the daughters (which can be read as descendants) are bound up in an ongoing history where they experience pain in the medical space that is often intangible and unquantifiable. The question is critical because repair depends on it. This is why Judd returns to the question over and over again in this text. I think of the unnamed victims of medical experimentation performed by Sims and other doctors of the time, those who weren't documented in the archive, those "misremembered and unaccounted for," as Toni Morrison's *Beloved* would have it.

I also think of the overwhelming numbers of unknown victims of medical experimentation in the name of gynecological and obstetric advancement when I am in Montgomery's Legacy Museum: From Slavery to Mass Incarceration—an excursion I took during the Anarcha Lucy Betsey Day of Reckoning Conference. The museum, which is located just blocks from one of the most prominent slave auction spaces in the United States, explores the history of transatlantic slavery and its contemporary legacies. As I toured the space, I came across an account describing an enslaved woman named Martha that made me pause: "Martha, about 36, good cook and plantation hand, smart woman and good character. Has been somewhat troubled recently with womb complaint, otherwise very healthy and strong, fair seamstress, and very handy." Here we see direct reference to the enslaved woman's womb as a key descriptor of her suitability for service. I am also intrigued by the resonance of the word *complaint*. Was this Martha's way of resisting? What are the multiple valences of complaint here? I held this story with me throughout my time in Montgomery. I kept thinking about Martha's womb complaint as I heard the contemporary stories during the conference of Black birthing people's womb complaints being ignored and disregarded. It was overwhelming. Thankfully, on my last day in Montgomery, I had additional time and was able to return to the Mothers of Gynecology Park to linger in the space of reflection (a space separate from the main areas) that Browder had created to contemplate all that I had seen and heard. Tucked back away from the statues and onlookers, the reflection space was a private sanctuary with benches and pillows as well as visual art and messages that invited respite from the harsh historical experiences one encounters all over the city. I sat there for about an hour thinking about all I had seen. It was there that I began to explore the questions racing through my own creative rememory work, the result of which follows:

Womb Complaint

Complaint—a statement that a situation is unsatisfactory or unacceptable.
Pain of the womb
Discomfort
The lost child
The taken child
It remembers; it complains
It protests its status as property
As it bears life to enter a living death
Unrealized potential
It is not compliant
It complains
It speaks on behalf of
Words that cannot be said aloud
Refusing its role in the production of racial capital
It complains, it protests,
It resists.

How does one measure this pain?

CREATIVITY AS RESISTANCE

The creative work and archival histories I encountered in Montgomery demonstrate how creativity and radical imagining can serve as disruptions to historical accounts that obscure or even attempt to erase Black voices. This work facilitates resistance and generates something new. In contemporary creatives who are working against the backdrop of painful histories and often responding to them, we can see a form of liberatory creativity emerge where they refuse to be bound by the pain of such histories or even defined by them. I saw this up close throughout communities in the Dallas and broader North Texas region in the lead-up to the undoing of *Roe v. Wade.*

There was a kind of electric energy in the air from 2021 to 2022, and the Reproductive Liberation rallies (led by the Afiya Center in partnership with Planned Parenthood of Greater Texas) became sites of collective healing, community rebuilding, and resistance. We were relearning how to be in shared space together because of Covid-19, but so much social upheaval (from the racial reckonings of 2020, to the tumult of the 2020 presidential election, to the attacks on bodily autonomy that targeted *Roe v. Wade* and gender-affirming surgeries for youth) made it impossible to remain isolated from one another. The uniqueness of these spaces was their irreverence. Fellow protesters danced, marched, and chanted together. "Fuck Greg Abbott" was a common refrain. The rallies eventually drew the attention of the media, where respectability politics became a cudgel to attack protesters.

An article on Breitbart.com entitled "Video: Women 'Twerking for Abortions' in Dallas as SCOTUS Overrules Roe. v. Wade" illustrates the kinds of backlash conservative commentators tried to incite against these liberatory demonstrations.[23] The article quoted various social media reactions that attacked protesters. On Twitter, Elijah Schaffer wrote, "Dallas women TWERKING for abortions WTF . . . 'Shakin dat a** so we can kill our babies, proud to be a hoe and not be a ladies.[*sic*]'" The responses to the Breitbart article, loaded with judgment and blame, mirrored Schaffer's. The commentators suggested that these kinds of displays were why antiabortion advocates couldn't take their opposition seriously. But what organizations like the Afiya Center know is

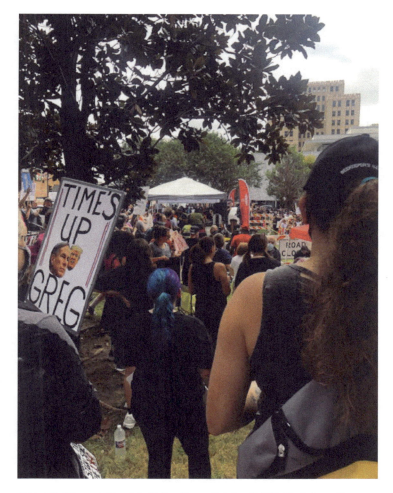

Figure 2. Women's March in Dallas, Texas, October 2, 2021. Photo by author.

that respectability politics won't save us and that people deserve to be sexually free without shame because at the heart of bodily autonomy is the right to decide what one does with one's body, especially with respect to sexuality—the most publicly maligned aspect of bodily freedom. The rally organizers were enacting what adrienne maree brown terms "pleasure activism," a mode of resistance that "is the work we do to reclaim our whole, happy, and satisfiable selves from the impacts, delusions, and limitations of oppression and/or supremacy."[24] At these reproductive freedom rallies, attendees were encouraged to embrace themselves unapologetically. So twerking was not just twerking. It was tapping into the generative force of pleasure to enact justice, healing, and collective liberation.

In many senses, the music, the twerking, and the gathering were performing aligned political work much like Michelle Browder's Anarcha Lucy Betsey Day of Reckoning. They were creating space to be free of the historical and present burdens of white supremacy and patriarchal harm, and to mourn and commune with all those affected by these harms. The approaches were just different. Daphne Brooks, in her *Liner Notes for the Revolution*, makes clear that "Black women's musical practices are, in short, revolutionary because they are inextricably linked to the matter of Black life."[25] Their practices both "forecast and execute the viability and potentiality of Black life." The music and movement that brought activists and community members together worked in the service of affirming Black life and reclaiming the narrative of what it means to be "prolife."

I think of the work of the Afiya Center and their allies as a kind of affective and sonic survival that is irreverent and unapologetic in its expressive posture. This work is an enactment of the "Black ratchet imagination" or "ratchetness as praxis" that thinkers Britney Cooper, L.H. Stallings, Bettina Love, and more theorize.[26] Coined in early 2000s hip-hop culture/vernacular, *ratchetness* describes someone who is unruly, "ghetto," sassy, or out of control in their behaviors. Cooper, Stallings, and Love, and other scholars, however, see the embrace of ratchetness

Rememory: A Reproductive Justice Mixtape / 89

as simultaneously a rejection of respectability politics, which, Cooper avers, "has failed Black women, and continues to disallow the access that we have been taught to think it will give."[27] She and Stallings invite us to think about what ratchetness itself makes possible and what the Black ratchet imagination might compel us to create. The question of what ratchetness makes possible is what I can imagine informs the practices of the Afiya Center and similar organizations that refuse to subscribe to the "perfect victim" discourse and instead embrace all those who need advocacy and who are unapologetically themselves. Their praxis involves a full-throated call for bodily autonomy, most critically the right to be sexually empowered and to be able to determine their futures. At their rallies, they create a site of freedom for all those attending. Crowds are diverse with respect to race, gender, and sexuality. Correspondingly, our playlist for the Livable Black Futures Collective expressed this ethos. As we were thinking together about what livable Black futures looked like, we were doing so to a soundtrack full of ratchet-affirming music.

One such song that became an anthem for us was Megan Thee Stallion's "Plan B." Released in April 2022, only months before the Supreme Court decided *Dobbs v. Jackson*, "Plan B" placed an exclamation point on our evolving playlist. Megan Thee Stallion's own journey to be heard after being a victim of unconscionable violence (she was shot in the foot by Torey Lanez in 2020),[28] as well as her Texas roots, resonated for us deeply because essentially she was performing a kind of storytelling work in public similar to what we were engaged in within our Livable Black Futures Storytelling Project. In 2020, two years preceding the release of "Plan B," Megan Thee Stallion was engaged in deep public advocacy for Black women and bodily autonomy. In October 2020, she offered a multipronged response to the various indignities and harms that

Black women, including herself, had recently experienced via her performance on *Saturday Night Live (SNL)* and an op-ed that she penned for the *New York Times*. On *Saturday Night Live*, she protested Kentucky attorney general Daniel Cameron's decision not to pursue criminal charges against the officers who had killed Breonna Taylor in her home in March 2020. Cameron ultimately only charged one officer, Brett Hankinson, for wanton endangerment over shooting into neighboring apartments.[29] This sparked widespread public outrage, which Megan channeled into her performance on *SNL*. She then followed up that performance with the publication of her *New York Times* op-ed entitled "Why I Speak Up for Black Women," where she proclaimed: "We [Black women] deserve to be protected as human beings. And we are entitled to our anger about a laundry list of mistreatment and neglect that we suffer."[30] She cited everything from the maternal mortality rates for Black mothers to the shaming of women who dress in unapologetically body-affirming ways. She asserted that "when women choose to capitalize on our sexuality, to reclaim our *own* power, like I have, we are vilified and disrespected." Reclaiming her power (and thereby inspiring others to reclaim theirs) became a deepened focus of her artistry.

For those of us in reproductive justice spaces, "Plan B" provided language for the act of taking back one's power after being disrespected and mistreated. Addressed to a composite figure in a relationship gone wrong, it is in many ways an anthem for bodily autonomy and self-determination. With lyrics highlighting the value of independence and self-worth that isn't bound up in others or systems, it is an empowering narrative for anyone who is rejecting oppressive conditions. Playing artists like Megan Thee Stallion and twerking at rallies are forms of bodily autonomy, irreverent protest, and embodied joy. They exhibit *ratchetness as a praxis* and pleasure activism, making new worlds possible through resistance. Attendees leave these rallies mobilized to reclaim their power and joy even as the state works actively to oppress them.

COLLECTIVE REMEMORY AND WATERBREAKING

The power of the creative and the imagination to mobilize communities became a centerpiece of the Livable Black Futures experience. Returning to the playlist concept that grounded our work, we also drew on various forms of literary expression as a tool to inspire our storytellers to harness the power of their voices and to tell their stories without shame. Just as the playlist constituted a mixtape for reproductive justice, the imaginative work we engaged added to what felt like a remix of stories and memories that resonated (and continue to resonate) across time and space. Like a palimpsest, our stories were layered onto one another's and onto histories—each time we pulled back a layer, we'd find resonance with a story from the past. To return to my concept of waterbreaking, the breaking of silences about experiences of trauma and pain via creative expression lent itself to an outpouring on behalf of the storytellers whose stories flowed from the narratives we were listening to and reading.

One particular work that facilitated the expressive community building we were engaged in was reelaviolette botts-ward's *mourning my inner [blackgirl] child*, a collection of poetry that reflects on everything from girlhood, to embodied memory, to ancestral grieving. This work grows out of botts-ward's community project called blackwomxnhealing.com, an online repository of various forms of artistic collectivity (from visual art forms such as collage, to poetry, to self-portraiture and more) among Black women who were working to heal in the wake of 2020, amid Covid-19 and the short-lived racial reckonings during this time. botts-ward modeled for us what collectivity could look like during and in the aftermath of the Covid-19 lockdown and its attendant isolation. So much of the collection spoke to our community because of its deep engagement with the work of mourning and healing, which were at the heart of our project. In her article "curating #blackgirlquarantine," botts-ward writes about how the project was meant to support Black women as they navigated their collective grief, including her own unhealed pain. In the production of the exhibit, botts-ward attended to various elements of cultural preservation that paralleled the work we saw coming forward in the Livable Black Futures Storytelling Project. She drew on sound as a form of healing, bringing forth the voice of Braxton, a member of the blackwomxnhealing community who had passed away on November 2, 2020, as a way to open the exhibit and ground it in an ancestral presence that would resonate across the images and experience overall. The blending of sound and image (the act of listening and seeing in a deeper way) corresponded with much of the work we were doing with our collective. It felt right, then, to blend botts-ward's poetry with ours.

On the last day of the first iteration of the Livable Black Futures storytelling circles, we read botts-ward's "Healing at Home: A Love Letter to Blackgirl Sanctuary," from *mourning my inner [blackgirl] child*. It spoke to the ways we were navigating our relationships to home: being between homes, moving, transitioning from houselessness to having a home, remodeling, and so on. "Healing at Home" is an ode to a living space, a space the speaker is working to make a home. It explores the ways we adjust to our environments in order to create a life. The poem also deepens this by meditating on the notion of interiority and vulnerability and a place where Black women can be themselves. At one point in the poem, the speaker asks, almost as proclamation:

> and don't every black woman deserve this,
> a space she can call her sanctuary?
> to sit still in her magic
> and make meaning of her life.[31]

We read aloud and discussed this poem together, and this line of questioning resonated with many in our group. It was essentially what we were in search of—Black girl sanctuary.

As we discussed the significance of botts-ward's words, we thought about the sanctuary we had found together. After our conversation, we picked lines that we wanted to hold onto. One of our doulas, D'Andra, talked about how the poem had helped her to describe the services they offered. Regarding botts-ward's line "And don't every Black woman deserve this?" D'Andra expressed that "every Black woman deserves a space, and a circle of sisterhood or genuine people who care and can relate to their experiences," a direct counter to feelings of unworthiness that many of our storytellers said that they had often felt.

In many ways, *mourning my inner [blackgirl] child* facilitated a waterbreaking for everyone engaging with her poetry. The poetry opened up a space for us to talk about how overall sexual and reproductive trauma as well as indignity had shaped much of how we saw ourselves and our worthiness. One storyteller spoke about navigating public assistance as a Black mother. She said she often felt treated like a criminal: "You almost have to give your blood [to receive help]. They want to do drug tests. You have to deny your relationship if you aren't married because a man can't live with you if you are receiving assistance. You can't have a co-parent. If you need affordable housing, you have to submit to inspections." For this storyteller, accepting public assistance meant not being able to have sanctuary and constantly being under the surveillance of the state.

State surveillance took on a deeper resonance because Texas was in the middle of passing Senate Bill 8, which not only sanctioned health care providers to report those suspected of having abortions but gave everyday individuals the charge to do so as well. So the conversation inevitably led to topics around safety and how to find a place where women could be their authentic selves. One storyteller offered: "For me, my home is my sanctuary. I pray to the sacred space; when I walk in my home, you can just feel the good energy. You can feel the relaxation. You can feel the peace, because to me, your house should be a place where you could go to, to find peace that you can't find in the world. And when the world beats you up, you should have a place that you can go to." The need to find sanctuary and hold sacred space for oneself was a topic that we lingered on for a good deal of time. With Covid-19 many of us had spent the last year isolating in our homes, so the stakes of home as a sanctuary felt higher too. Some storytellers even expanded on how they had created sanctuary in their homes but also worked to build community with others experiencing isolation. Such work included a resource group for women who relied on public assistance and a conversation platform hosted on YouTube where Black women across generations could talk openly and share their experiences on a range of topics that included sexual and reproductive health. These storytellers were finding ways to facilitate their own safety in an increasingly unsafe context.

Safety for Black birthing people in health care spaces is not guaranteed. In their essay "Emotional Safety Is Patient Safety," Audrey Lyndon, Dána-Ain Davis, Anjana E. Sharma, and Karen A.

Scott explain the importance of patient safety for Black patients, asserting: "We fully endorse the need for changing the paradigm in patient safety."[32] There is a need to bridge the gap between hospitals' protocols that underlie patients' being safe and patient experiences of "feeling safe." To do this, Lyndon et al. affirm, "A more expansive and inclusive definition of harm within the existing safety paradigm must recognize and act upon the reality that dismissal, disrespect, abuse, class bias, ableism, fatphobia, racism, sexism, and transphobia in healthcare all exemplify failure to see patients as whole human beings who are experts on their own bodies and experiences, deserving of dignity and respect."[33] Without this expansive understanding of patient harm, patient safety remains elusive.

The storytellers' desires to invest in their own sanctuary spaces and in their safety must also be understood within the context of their generational traumas. Many of them reported their mothers and grandmothers passing away at early ages or contending with health issues across the span of their lives. One storyteller recalled her mother's own history of pregnancy loss and poor health, which affected her so much she held great anxiety about carrying her own children to term. She said,

> I had to keep telling myself—your story is not your mama's story. It's not just me who struggles. My sister too. She had a baby a couple months ago and was diagnosed with high blood pressure. Now she has this anxiety, and it's like, she thinks that she's going to die like our mama. I have to keep telling her, you are not mama. But it's hard. I remember when I had my last miscarriage, I was relieved. Because I was like, I ain't got to worry about that happening now. I ain't got to deal with it now, you know what I'm saying? Like, and it was like, I lost the baby like the day before the anniversary, the twentieth anniversary of her passing. So I'm just like, there's so much going on. I mean, like emotionally just tore up, you know what

I'm saying? Like I'm definitely, I just keep . . . Allison [social worker] always telling me to speak positive things to myself. Because I have a tendency to try that, always saying, this can happen and that can happen, and this can happen. I'm always trying to come up with a plan B, C, D for everything in my life, which has me all over the place.

But I still haven't been oh, like telling myself every day, oh, you are beautiful, you are strong, you this, this and that. All I keep telling myself every day now, is I'm not my mama. I'm not going to die like my mama, my story is not hers. And I'm just, I'm feeling good about that. I mean, I still have some stuff I'm going with, dealing with, but that's the biggest part of me to say that no. Because I truly believe that, that's not my story. That's not going to happen to me.

This story demonstrates the multilayered and palimpsestic nature of stories of medical trauma and harm. It became apparent to me that the individuals sharing their stories with us brought whole histories into the space and were shaped by those experiences. Taking her cue from one of our storytellers, another storyteller proclaimed that her mother's story would not be hers as well. She was older, in her seventies, but she expressed that this was the first time she had shared with others the weight she had carried trying not to live out her mother's story and repeat that history. She shared, "My mom was forty-seven when she died, and she died too of a stroke and had blood pressure. I told myself, baby, I wouldn't do that. It was a wasted life. It was something, to me, that could have been prevented, but she was so angry and she died at forty-seven. I am seventy-four. And I lived to [my] seventies, because I said it would not happen to me."

mourning my inner [blackgirl] child helped our storytellers voice the many layers of their journey to support themselves in a world where that is not a given. Their observations resonated with me, as did the need to account for generational trauma in our conversations about sexual and reproductive health. I lingered on this passage from "Healing at Home" that speaks to Alice Walker's work to amplify the inner lives of our mothers and grandmothers, as well as how to reconcile the pain of the past with the wisdom it provides:

> that day at the meditation center
> alice walker reminded me
> with her soft hands and calm smile
> embracing me carefully
> *"you have the power, sister"*
>
> the power to cultivate a garden
> to pull from the powers of my mothers
> to pull from the depths of the dirt
> and dig out the gem
> to know that light always wins
> and i will always be light so long as i choose
> and now i am light
> and now you are light too.[34]

In the constellation of our experiences, there is individual and collective power. This power is bound up in our mothers, place, and the broader energy of the universe. We shared that energy and bonded through it through our creativity—our light. Through our stories we were able to cast light—to radiate and illuminate in ways that we had not done before and could not do without each other. Much like botts-ward, who used collage as a tool for materializing the collectivity of Black women, we created a collage born from unhealed trauma and our determination to recover.

AFTERMEMORY

Bettina Judd's *patient* includes a poem called "After Memory." The poem riffs off Lucille Clifton's "why some people be mad at me sometimes," where she writes:

they ask me to remember
but they want me to remember
their memories
and i keep on remembering
mine.[35]

Clifton highlights how the act of remembering is not neutral. Often there is a contest for whose story takes precedence, whose version of events is seen as valid. When we insist on telling the truth of our memories, no matter how hard these truths are, people often respond in anger. This is a confirmation of the power of memory and the act of remembering on the part of those who are vulnerable and often marginalized. Judd contemplates what happens after memory. Whose stories get preserved, and what narratives are privileged over others? Judd's poem reads:

> It's like when a black person says: "that's racist!" to a white person and they refuse to believe. Maybe it is better to say, "This moment is steeped in a racist history. This racist history is indelibly printed on my memory. You do not want to remember, so you wish to erase mine." But it is not heard. One only hears what one hopes not to be, and that's racist.
>
> After memory, I am absent. No table. No one on all fours. No children living or otherwise. No hymns. No nursemaids. No sideshow freaks. No experiments. No spoon. No bent handle, no wincing. Just whiskey, opium and: *Now, wasn't there some good?*[36]

Judd details the cost of what happens after memory—after the stories are told and not held. These histories are in danger of being erased and sanitized in favor of the oppressor's narrative. Wasn't there some good that came out of all this pain? But this is not the question we need to ask. In fact, this is a harmful question because it reframes one's trauma and uses whatever scientific or cultural development came from it as a justification for the horrendous acts (in the case of Judd's poem, the brutal experimentations on enslaved women, the demeaning displays of Joice Heth and Saartjie Baartman, the exploitation of Henrietta Lacks's cells).

Judd frames "after memory" in temporal terms, as in what happens to memory after it has been released into the world and has been subsequently reframed and virtually erased. However, the Livable Black Futures experience offers another take on "after memory," or rather what I'd like to think of as "aftermemory"—the result of sharing one's memories in supportive community and with those who are invested in holding space for you and your stories. I think of it as a play on both Morrison's concept of "rememory" and "afterbirth" (the expelling of the placenta after the baby has been delivered). To me, "aftermemory" is the residue of releasing painful memories—those inside you that you have to nurse individually through the placenta of your inner life. When we release those memories into the world, we hold them up to others for them to also see and reckon with. We no longer need to provide them with just our oxygen—bearing them in our silence. When we tell our stories with intention and to those who desire to preserve them, we are engaging in aftermemory work. I think of Michelle Browder's *Mothers of Gynecology* statues, Megan Thee Stallion's vulnerable memory sharing after being assaulted with a deadly weapon, and reelaviolette botts-ward's blackwomxnhealing work, which is about remembering those who have passed away. Aftermemory has a generative capacity, much like waterbreaking. The two concepts can be read alongside each other as a vernacular of Black storytelling. It is how we carry history forward, how we reckon with it, and how we heal.

CHAPTER FOUR

Imagining Livable Black Futures

Affirmation
I imagine futures for myself and Black people that are livable, free, and just.

We are in an imagination battle.

—adrienne maree brown

What can we imagine for ourselves and the world?

—Mariame Kaba

Imagination has played a critical role in my journey to create space for Black women and birthing people to share their stories and to be held in loving community; in fact, I couldn't have done this work without it. In rememory and in the generative force of Black feminist creativity, imagination is key to moving from memory and toward possible futures. I am particularly thinking about the Black radical imagination, which involves both imagining a world without oppression and understanding mechanisms that produce subjection and working to dismantle them. This is the Black radical imagination that Robin D.G. Kelley speaks of in his work *Freedom Dreams*. Kelley sees creative expressive forces like Black poetry, Afrofuturism, and Afrosurrealism as inextricably linked to social movement work. He cites Charia Rose, who says, "If it weren't for the simple fact of imagining a future that could be non-oppressive ... then we wouldn't be in the streets or changing things within government or creative fields."[1] He also stresses that the Black radical imagination isn't a dream state but is instead forged in collective movements.[2] It is a marrying of theory with practice. Thinkers such as Assata Shakur make the point that theory without practice is just as incomplete as practice without theory. Because I am primarily a literary scholar, my research is based in analyses of literature and Black expressive culture. Thus for me imagination serves as a key entry point for moving from the theory work of Black imagining to its application in the world. Endarkened storywork[3] is a form of creating the future that we want to see.

My work is also rooted in a deep personal history of ancestral imagining, one that I witnessed in my own upbringing. The Black ancestors in my life were constantly imagining better worlds despite oppressive conditions. Living in Mississippi amid extensive poverty, oppression, and racial terror in the twentieth century meant having to believe in the unimaginable and in something not yet seen. Kelley makes clear that our historical movements (from slavery to the present) have been grounded in "trying to sustain life by beating back the death-dealing structures of gendered racial capitalism. The only way to ensure survival for Black people was to envision a radically different future for all and fight to bring it into existence."[4] When I was growing up in rural Mississippi in the post–civil rights and Reagan eras, freedom dreams and imagination were often all my family had. My grandmothers would invite me to imagine all that I could be in this world every chance they got. Never mind that neither of them had made it past the sixth grade; they let me know that anything was possible for me. It was a mixture of faith and Black radical imagination.

My investment in imaginative work is also informed by the "Black ratchet imagination" (as L.H. Stallings terms it) and by other scholars' exploration of the creative and imaginative work of Black women rap artists and culture bearers, which offers possibilities for freedom beyond the shackles of respectability politics. The Livable Black Futures Collective is guided by these various forms of Black imagining for freedom. In this chapter, I reflect on how critical Black radical imagination has been for me as a scholar and community advocate and how I drew on it to support our Livable Black Futures storytellers to imagine liberated futures for themselves and for Black people. From thinkers such as Audre Lorde and adrienne maree brown, as well as the knowledge producers of the Livable Black Futures Storytelling Project, we can see how Black storytelling for reproductive justice pushes us from our precarious present to otherwise imagining (building community and cocreating our futures) and serves as a form of strategizing in oppressive times. Envisioning future possibilities offers us paths to surviving and thriving in our present and beyond. Reproductive justice is animated by freedom dreams and is a key example of this concept.

RADICAL IMAGINING

Audre Lorde's 1979 essay "Man Child: A Black Lesbian Feminist's Response" is a powerful meditation on mothering and its potential connection to liberation. For Lorde, the two are deeply intertwined. Rather than take the posture of expert, she details her process of learning and loving out loud as she works to support her children in an anti-Black world. The essay contemplates how she must mother in order to ensure that her children survive beyond her. It focuses on her son Jonathan (fifteen years old at the time of her writing). Lorde notes that he faces unique challenges growing up as a Black boy, soon to be a man, and being raised by two lesbian women in the 1970s, a time when the effects of the civil rights movement still linger but when Black and queer equality feels very distant. She writes, "Raising black children—male and female—in the mouth of a racist, sexist, suicidal dragon is perilous and chancy."[5] Thus mothers must teach them to love and resist at the same time in order to survive.

Lorde contemplates the future, and while she holds freedom dreams for her children, her central goal is that their lives are livable and that they survive. She says, "When I envision the future, I think of the world I crave for my daughters and my sons. It is thinking for the survival of the species—thinking for life."[6] What I appreciate here is Lorde's deeply held perspective that when basic needs such as safety and social support are absent for Black children, freedom dreams sometimes look like simply surviving to see the future. This piece reminds me that this is not something Black people can take for granted, and Lorde develops this line of thought compellingly through the viewpoint of a Black mother. The essay aligned closely with what I had been reading about reproductive justice and its central tenets: the right to have children; the right not to have children; and the right to nurture the children we have in a safe and healthy environment. While these feel like basic rights, they are not rights that are guaranteed to all. This is why Lorde says, "As a black woman committed to a livable future, and as a mother loving and raising a boy who will become a man, I must examine all my possibilities for being within such a destructive system."[7] Lorde's words raise the question: What does a livable Black future look like now? She spends time naming the 1970s context of what livable futures look like—resisting white supremacist ideals, fighting back against sexism, and advocating for racial and gender equality. While her framing is not too distant from the contemporary challenges facing Black people, I was curious about how, through storytelling, we might name what a livable future is in the precarious present (amid Covid-19, attacks on gender-affirming care and abortion, growing transphobia and homophobia, anti-Black police violence, and more) during which I was embarking on this research. So Lorde's essay became foundational to our research question, *What does a livable Black future look like now?*

The question is an interdisciplinary and intersectional one. Thinkers such as Audre Lorde bring to bear multiple knowledges that responding to it requires. Responding to this question demands a blend of activist theorizing and radical love, both of which Black feminist leaders have offered us across time. For them, Black mothering has always been political.[8] In addition to Lorde, I think of Ida B. Wells, who would breastfeed her infant children while on the lynching lecture circuit. Wells wrote beautiful letters to her children while away, especially when she had to miss a holiday. I am taken by one in particular in her archives where she has to miss Halloween and tells her children how much she loves them and how wonderful they are.[9] She writes to them, "Whenever I think of my dear girls, which is all the time, such a feeling of confidence comes over me. I know my girls are true to me, to themselves and to their God wherever they are, and my heart is content." While Wells is lauded often for her activism, this work of mothering is also a critical part of her legacy. She took great pride in her children and lifted them up in spite of the contexts in which they lived. To care for her children during a time where Black death was treated as a casual occurrence and a spectacle is to resist the oppressive forces hoping to render Blackness as a social death. This is also true for Fannie Lou Hamer, who discussed openly her desire to become a mother even after the state of Mississippi sterilized her without her knowledge. In spite of this attempt to render her childless, Fannie Lou Hamer would go on to adopt four children—Dorothy Jean, Vergie Ree, Lenora Aretha, and Jacqueline Denise (she would also periodically care for her husband Pap's daughter Linnie). Both Fannie Lou Hamer and Ida B. Wells were admonished, largely by white women activists, not to pursue motherhood because it would sap their energies for their activist work. Each woman dismissed this advice, citing the import of motherhood for them as Black women.[10] They, too, were committed to creating livable Black futures for their children and all Black children.

Thinkers and activists like Lorde, Wells, and Hamer have served as embodiments of the work of freedom dreams. The creative is another space where Black women have charted a vision for the future rooted in Black viability. Octavia Butler is one writer who harnessed the power of creativity to advance possibility in an anti-Black and sexist world. Her novel *Parable of the Sower* explicitly demonstrates this. It is a form of future imagining that is foundationally Black affirming. Published in 1993, *Parable of the Sower* is set in the 2020s in an apocalyptic California where social chaos reigns because of climate change, economic crises, and political upheaval. In many ways, Butler anticipates the precarious era that has been the 2020s, with Covid-19 exacerbating issues of health and mental wellness, as well as exposing to a broader world various systemic racial and gender inequalities that led to the uprisings of 2020.

At the heart of the work is a Black girl—fifteen-year-old Lauren Olamina, who suffers from hyperempathy, a debilitating sensitivity to others' emotions. As she faces the challenge of losing her family members and having to forge her future alone, Lauren joins with others and leads them on a journey that is both a fight for survival and a birthing of a new faith, Earthseed. Along the way, she meets a man who will eventually become her husband. His name is Bankole, and he is a Black doctor working to return to his three-hundred-acre farm in Mendocino and reunite with his sister and larger family who are living there. The novel keeps returning to Lauren's refrain as one of the only constants of life:

> All that you touch
> You Change.
>
> All that you Change
> Changes you.
>
> The only lasting truth
> Is Change.
>
> God
> Is Change.[11]

We can think of this poem as a theory of change guided by interdependence, most critically theorized by Audre Lorde. Refusing to acknowledge the constancy of change and our interconnectedness only leads to a world of violence, oppression, and chaos. Butler offers us a different future. With Lauren, a Black disabled woman, at the center of the work, we understand that (as the Combahee River Collective proclaims) freeing Black women means dismantling all systems of oppression.

adrienne maree brown builds on this theory of change and creates a holistic vision for what she calls "emergent strategies." She defines emergent strategies as "how we intentionally change in ways that grow our capacity to embody the just and liberated worlds we long for."[12] brown's vision is guided by the notion that since change is inevitable, we must be strategic in the process in order to create transformative futures. Butler is a compass for brown. She writes: "Octavia Butler, one of the cornerstones of my awareness of emergent strategy, spoke of the fatal human flaw as a combination of hierarchy and intelligence. We are brilliant at survival, but brutal at it. We tend to slip out of togetherness the way we slip out of the womb, bloody and messy and surprised to be alone. And clever—able to learn with our bodies the ways of this world."[13] brown seeks a world where the future is created with our interdependence in mind—a world with principles of dignity, collective power, love, generative conflict, and community at its heart. Imagination is key to making such a future possible. brown notes, "A visionary exploration of humanity includes imagination. Octavia spent her life working through complex ideas of the future on behalf of humans."[14] These words echo the words of Lucille Clifton: "We cannot create what we can't imagine." Imagination is the force for change. When we tap into the creative power of imagining, we are breaking free from the world that is and moving toward the world we dream of. More than that, there are high stakes to the work of imagining. adrienne maree brown captures this compellingly when she writes: "We are in an imagination battle. Trayvon Martin and Mike Brown and Renisha McBride and so many others are dead because, in some white imagination, they were dangerous. And that imagination is so respected that those who kill, based on an imagined, racialized fear of Black people, are rarely held accountable."[15] She calls this work a "time-travel exercise for the heart" and a collaborative ideation. brown shows the life-and-death consequences of imagination. This was why it was important to end our Livable Black Futures

Storytelling experience with an exercise of imagining what livable Black futures looked like for Black birthing people.

Early on in our time together, we asked our storytellers what came to mind when they heard the phrase "livable Black futures" and what it meant for each of us. Storytellers offered up the following: determination, safe, free, proud, being able to just "be," unapologetic, fearless, nonjudgmental, agency, community, being heard, joy, seeing, and peace. As they offered up the words, we wrote them on sheets of paper placed on the walls of our meeting room so that we could see them throughout our experience and start to think about what it would look like to create the world where all those words are the texts of Black life instead of the precarity that hovers over the concept of Black life. At the end of our time, we returned to these words to create what we would call a "Black Wombholders' Bill of Rights." We felt that if we started there, the principles of having a livable Black future would materialize beyond our experiences with sexual and reproductive health.

THE BLACK WOMBHOLDERS' BILL OF RIGHTS

The creation of a community-based Bill of Rights is an act of imagination and empowerment for individuals who are often left out of the deliberative process for determining what their rights should be. We aimed to construct a rhetorically powerful document that could amplify the voices of our storytellers and be an effective advocacy tool. In producing our Bill of Rights, we relied on effective models from allies who were doing similar work. One such model was the Community Bill of Rights drawn up by the Full Frame Initiative, an alliance of government, community, and nonprofit change makers who are working to challenge oppressive systems such as racism, homophobia, sexism, and additional inequalities so that everyone has a "fair shot at well-being."[16] According to the Initiative, "Centering community is a practice that allows for social justice efforts to build the durable solutions needed to address . . . systemic problems [the systemic injustices individuals endure while navigating institutions and services]. The Community Bill of Rights provides the necessary steps for systems to reach those solutions." The process of looking to community for possible solutions to the challenges we face is something that the Afiya Center values inherently. The Center serves the community and seeks to employ and engage community members so that their voices are not lost in these conversations. So our production of the Black Wombholders' Bill of Rights spoke directly to these values. We also looked to existing patient bills of rights produced in community. One central model was the National Association to Advance Black Birth and their "Black Birthing Bill of Rights."[17] We found this document to be an effective tool to name the principles that support Black birthing people throughout their pregnancies. The rights they list include statements like "I have the right to be listened to and heard," "I have the right to have my humanity acknowledged," and "I have the right to choose how I want to nourish my child and have my choice be supported." This document reflected our goal to create a document that would offer similar kinds of empowering statements; however, we wanted to expand the conversation beyond birth, given that we had uncovered a range of gynecological and obstetric harms as well as issues within our communities that needed to be addressed.

The Black Wombholders' Bill of Rights is an in-process document that we see expanding as we continue to advance conversations about Black sexual and reproductive health. The following details the drafting process and the wide range of conversations we had as we produced the document. The in-process document is offered after this narrative of our deliberation process. I have organized the conversation into topics that emerged, and I offer a representation of the comments that aligned with each idea. We all agreed that the process of creating this bill of rights felt restorative and empowering. We also drew on imagination as a tool and took the approach of demanding the impossible, a strategy used in justice movements to name the world we want to see—not the world as it is.

The Right to Have or Not Have Children

Our conversation immediately turned to the central tenet of reproductive justice—the right to have children and the right *not* to have children—given the contemporary realities we were facing with Senate Bill 8 in Texas (also known as "the Heartbeat Bill"),[18] which bans abortion after six weeks into pregnancy, the time when legislators claim a fetal heartbeat can be detected—effectively banning abortion almost entirely. This law also endorses vigilante acts such as surveillance and even violence by its reliance on civil enforcement through lawsuits.[19] The constitutionality of such acts is being challenged through various legal channels, but during our gathering, the threat of this kind of surveillance was (and remains) a deep concern, especially because Black people are often subject to surveillance in various contexts and criminalized. More than that, the prospect of forced pregnancy constitutes a rewinding of the clock for Black people in matters of bodily autonomy. It feels like slavery by another name. One storyteller described the challenge of being pregnant and in a harmful relationship. "You're having to deal with other things that you really don't want to fucking deal with. When you realize you may be pregnant in two months and you think to yourself, 'I really don't like this man that much.'"

Feelings of being stuck in a partnership because of pregnancy were very prevalent in the room. Many of the storytellers had already encountered challenges to receiving an abortion even before Senate Bill 8 became law. They described going to crisis pregnancy centers (CPCs) and being discouraged from having an abortion. The harms of crisis pregnancy centers are increasingly being documented, particularly their practices of being purposefully manipulative and spreading misinformation about pregnancy and abortion.[20] One of our storytellers expressed concern that she was misled that her pregnancy was actually terminated. She ended up giving birth in the months following her visit.

Throughout this conversation, fear was a predominant emotion. Storytellers felt very concerned that they were seeing their reproductive autonomy being stripped away before their eyes, and they felt powerless to stop it. Our community was one safe place to express these concerns and to name them in the Wombholders' Bill of Rights.

Informed Consent

In addition to concerns about abortion access and fertility management, storytellers felt underserved when it came to engagement with providers and patient education. They remarked that most providers spent very little time with them during visits—leaving them feeling unheard. One storyteller stated, "I feel like we have the right to be educated. Don't just present things to me without explaining. Tell me the effects of the Depo shot. Educate me about my options so that I can be informed." This resonated with many in the room, especially given the history of sterilization that many Black birthing people have endured. One such fertility-disrupting agent is the Depo Provera shot and others like it, namely Norplant—essentially forms of temporary sterilization. Scholars such as Dorothy Roberts in *Killing the Black Body* have recounted how these shots have been administered through coercive measures to poor Black mothers and teenagers as a condition of receiving benefits and often at the expense of their health, with documented harms including irregular and prolonged heavy bleeding, muscle weakness, and even fatal hemorrhaging.[21] Given the risks, providers need to spend more time discussing these concerns with patients. Our storytellers cited this as a chief issue when determining birth control methods as a form of family planning.

More organic and natural forms of birth control were also desired. One storyteller asked, "How about the right to be educated on the choices for birth control from natural, herbal medicines, surgical?" This question led to a discussion about medicine's hostility to holistic health practices, which often leaves many birthing people lacking many options for birth control. This was something our storytellers wanted to receive more information on when making decisions about contraceptives.

Shame- and Stigma-Free Conversations

The conversation on shame and stigma was central to the storytelling experience. Early on in our time together, many storytellers reported that their silence was often a product of shame and stigma experienced within their communities and at the doctor's office. Many storytellers reported feeling morally judged at crisis pregnancy centers and in health care spaces generally. One person stated: "Don't project your morals onto me. So I have the right to a judgment-free experience with a health care provider and a no-questions-asked abortion." Many storytellers responded in agreement that they felt judged for various reasons while seeking medical care, whether because they were a single parent, or were living with HIV, or simply did not want to be pregnant yet wanted to be sexually active.

In response to the many examples raised about stigma and shame, someone said, "Be un-fuckin'-apologetic. Because it just may be one person who may need to know at that very moment that it's okay. Like, I feel empowered now because you said it, because you actually told your truth." We all nodded in agreement. So many of us in seeing the power of our collectivity were witnessing firsthand the importance of breaking the silence on sexual and reproductive health. Our chief goal was to make this experience available to those beyond our group.

For our formerly incarcerated storytellers, the conversation included issues of sexual assault. Though sexual assault was not a concern exclusive to our formerly incarcerated storytellers, it was the one that dominated our conversations. Many of our storytellers discussed how prevalent sexual assault is, yet how much silence exists around it. A storyteller shared, "So my thing to you [other people in the room] is, however you need to get it out. I mean, talk about it and tell somebody. Also, when in sexual assaults and things like that, if you have contracted any type of infection, some infections lead to other things." There were so many layers of shame to navigate, and we felt it was imperative to create safe, judgment-free spaces we could talk about these issues.

One important aspect of silencing was that many of our formerly incarcerated storytellers were concerned about being met with retaliation if they spoke honestly about their experiences.

Many storytellers were currently on parole and nervous to challenge the system by sharing their concerns with lawmakers. Some of them could not vote. One storyteller asked, "If we cannot vote, how can we make our voices heard?" They felt that any complaint would put them at risk for being targeted and reimprisoned. One storyteller expressed fear of speaking up because of fear of never getting their child back from foster care. These very real concerns were also barriers to feeling heard and being further stigmatized.

Resource Support

Underlying our conversations was the matter of resource support and poverty. As mentioned earlier, people who receive government assistance or seek help do so at the expense of their dignity and agency. Their private lives are interrogated and they face judgment for their choices. One of our facilitators, D'Andra, emphasized that health care could not be discussed in isolation: "Poverty, food deserts, all this other stuff, lack of access to safe health care overall. I can't talk about one and not talk about the other. We have to have interconnected conversations. I can't show up and talk about abortion without talking about systemic racism." Here she highlighted that all these issues are intertwined and that without resources and support, Black birthing people are further marginalized.

One storyteller offered: "People are often forced to do risky things for food (sex work, theft, etc.), and when you do seek help, you are subject to judgment." We discussed how many of us knew folks who had been so desperate that they would do dangerous things to live. People also said that many do this because they feel there is nowhere to turn. Thus we have to create supportive spaces where people can receive the resources they need without strings attached. This includes mental health resources. So many of us were in the process of healing without having access to culturally responsive, qualified mental health practitioners. One storyteller stated, "The thing about it is I want a trauma doctor that looks like me." Thankfully, in our storytelling experience we drew on the expertise and mental health support of Dr. Allison Tomlinson, but we acknowledged that there needed to be a more robust form of mental health support for Black women and birthing people.

Gender-Expansive Sex Education

The conversations about shame and stigma led to issues of sexuality and sexism with regard to sexual and reproductive health. We had been grappling with the bans such as "Don't say gay" in Florida[22] and the increasing legislation against gender-affirming care for youth in our own state of Texas.[23] We recognized not only that these efforts violated the rights of those who are LGBTQ+ but also that they produced further silencing of queer sexual and reproductive health experiences. A storyteller offered, "Reproductive health is not just a responsibility of cis-women and not just for women. It's also for transgender men. They still have wombs and have to go to the gynecologist." By this time in our experience, we had engaged in deep conversations about queerness thanks to the diversity of our group, so we knew we needed to include language that dealt with indignities queer folk often experience in health care, such as misgendering, misnaming, and a general exclusion from medical spaces such as gynecologists' offices. One queer storyteller stated that it was important to demystify assumptions about pregnancy with regard to queer folks. She shared,

> When I came out to my aunt, she cried and I asked her, "Why are you crying? I'm okay." But she said she was crying because she didn't think that I would have children or get married. She didn't think that somebody being queer could have these things in life, and now she gets to see me live, right? My truth in my life, which is everything.... We need to create new images of what family, success, and motherhood looks like. We have to create the realities we deserve.

The call to "create the realities we deserve" resonated with many. In our collective sharing of the kinds of rights we deserved and the way we thought we should be treated in health care spaces, it felt like we were doing just that.

We also recognized the sexism inherent in the treatment of sex education in our culture. Women and girls are often made responsible to learn about sexual and reproductive health, particularly how not to get pregnant. Often boys and men do not have critical knowledges because education about menstrual cycles and other reproductive health issues is rarely directed at them. "It has to be for everybody," one storyteller said. "We can't keep making it just for folks who go bear the babies. It's got to be for everybody, and it has to start early. And we should bring our sons in on that." There was collective agreement that these conversations needed to be had outside of heteronormative contexts overall.

Care and Dignity

Our discussion of the need for tangible financial and structural support turned to support for mental well-being. We all recognized that if we were to be advocates, we would have to be mindful of the need to care for ourselves. Here we had the words of Audre Lorde in mind: "Caring for myself is not self-indulgence, it is self-preservation, and that is an act of political warfare."[24] We thought critically about what that meant for us. We had built an ethic of care into the experience, but what would it mean for us to practice care beyond our shared storytelling space? What would it mean to receive the kind of care that we deserved when we went to hospitals and doctor's visits? Our doulas, Qiana, D'Andra, and Helen, felt this deeply. Qiana said: "We have to support ourselves, especially those of us who are doulas and working in the community. We are not just offering training on sexual and reproductive health, but also supporting people's wellness. We have to be well ourselves." What would it mean to be well?

We also discussed the intersection between community care and self-care. Mariame Kaba has stated, "I don't believe in self-care: I believe in collective care, collectivizing our care, and thinking more about how we can help each other."[25] Kaba's words offer insight into our broader understanding of care, that our wellness is bound up in the community and that if our community is unwell, then so are we. This also works in the other direction. If we, as community members, are unwell, then we cannot do the critical work to support and advocate what we desire.

The Resulting Document

The following is the collective document we produced—the Black Wombholders' Bill of Rights, articulating in a comprehensive way all the things that came from our conversation. This document is a work in progress, but it reflects the sentiments of our group. We all resolved to have conversations about it and build on it.

Black Wombholders' Bill of Rights

- I have the right to choose *not* to have children at any point in my life.
- I have the unlimited right to an abortion at any gestational point in the pregnancy.
- I have the right to a judgment-free experience with health care providers and judgment-free conversations about sexual and reproductive health in my community.
- I have the right to a safe and compassionate gynecological health care experience.
- I have the right to receive information about *all* of the options available to me as they relate to my sexual and reproductive health.
- I have the right to make the best choice for me at *any* age!
- I have the right to care that is not informed by ableism or race-based medicine.
- I have the right to gynecological care that is not influenced by homophobia, transphobia, or any other normative perspective that does not consider my identity.
- I have the right to be called by my chosen name and not my given name during medical appointments.
- I have the right for my son to receive a thorough education on his sexual and reproductive health and rights.
- I have the right to supportive, shame-free, and antisexist community conversations about my sexual and reproductive health.
- I have the right for my voice to be heard free from retaliation.

The Black Wombholders' Bill of Rights has become a living document that we utilize in presentations on the work of the Livable

Black Futures Storytelling Project. With each iteration of the presentation, we gain additional suggestions for the Bill of Rights. We encourage audiences to interact with it and to consider how it can be an advocacy tool going forward. This statement was produced with an abolitionist ethos that requires imagining new possibilities. Mariame Kaba says,

> Being intentionally in relation to one another, a part of a collective, helps to not only imagine new worlds, but also to imagine ourselves differently.... Let's begin our abolitionist journey not with the question "What do we have now, and how can we make it better?" Instead, let's ask "What can we imagine for ourselves and the world?" If we do that, then boundless possibilities of a more just world await us.[26]

The Black Wombholders' Bill of Rights is an abolitionist document at its heart. Through what some might call "impossible" demands and lofty goals, it reflects our participation in the imagination battle that adrienne maree brown speaks of. It is a battle that we are determined to win.

CHAPTER FIVE

Abolition Medicine

Affirmation

"We are pregnant with freedom. We are a conspiracy."

For true, from the long end
of the looking glass, it appears

isolation is one way to quell
a revolution.

> —DaMaris B. Hill, "Truth Is a Mirror in the Hands of God: Assata in 1976"

I'm gonna live as hard as i can and as full as i can until i die. And i'm not letting these parasites, these oppressors, these greedy racist swine make me kill my children in my mind, before they are even born.

> —Assata Shakur, *Assata*

Reading Assata Shakur's political autobiography *Assata* gave me language for what it means to live free while bound. At the heart of the work is imaginative resistance akin to the imagination battle that adrienne maree brown references when considering the fictive narratives that inform stereotypes of blackness. Tracing her coming of age and her life as a political prisoner in the New York and New Jersey penal systems, *Assata* is an account of Shakur's resistance to what was essentially an attempt to kill her spirit and that of her comrades agitating for a better world for Black people in the post–civil rights era. In an ultimate act of imaginative resistance, Shakur became pregnant while imprisoned. Shakur details her experience conceiving her daughter Kakuya in 1974 with her codefendant and comrade Kamau Sadiki, just outside of the surveillance of the prison guards and to their dismay. This act of freedom was a reminder that the state's power over her body could only go so far—and that even deeply oppressed subjects have the capacity to resist. The conceiving of her daughter was not accidental for Assata but rather intentional. She saw her unjust incarceration as an attempt to foreclose any possibilities for her life. Imprisonment, like slavery, places an individual in a state of social death[1] with limited affective relations to people. Seeing this, Assata refused their efforts to isolate her from her relationships, and she fought intensely for the survival of her unborn child. It is this act that animates *We are Pregnant with Freedom*.

Perhaps no story better illustrates the legacies of the objectification of the Black body and its surveillance by the state during slavery and beyond than *Assata*. The book also shows how medicine and the state can often intertwine, creating the need to disentangle carceral logics from medicine, a process that many have named *abolition medicine*. Abolition medicine is a practice of interrogating the foundational carceral logics of health care as well as structural inequalities that reproduce health inequity. In addition to interrogating systemic social challenges that health care reproduces, abolition medicine encourages health care practitioners and institutions to use their social power to address underlying causes of health inequity: education, economic inequality, police brutality, mass incarceration, mental health, and health care access.[2] Carceral logics and inequality (racial, economic, gender, etc.) still shape the way Black reproduction is managed in hospitals and is even greater demonstrated in the care or lack of care for incarcerated Black birthing people. This chapter puts various narrative accounts of carceral medicine in conversation (those of Black writers, creatives, and the storytellers of the Livable Black Futures project) to show how medicine is enacted on the most vulnerable in ways that are not altogether distinct from the carceral logics underpinning mainstream health care. Their collective stories of struggle and resistance powerfully demonstrate the urgency of abolition medicine.

Assata Shakur's imaginative resistance helps us envision what abolition medicine can look like. In what I consider a poetic meditation and theory, Assata Shakur writes the poem "Love" as a reflection on her unborn child:

> Love is a contraband in Hell,
> cause love is acid
> that eats away bars.
>
> But you, me, and tomorrow
> hold hands and make vows
> that struggle will multiply.
>
> The hacksaw has two blades.
>
> The shotgun has two barrels.
>
> We are pregnant with freedom.
>
> We are a conspiracy.[3]

Love is a relational act that brings people together. It was one of the central things that the state most desired to take away from Assata. Isolating her away from society and her loved ones was a direct attempt to diminish her spirit. Her investment in love and her aligning of her pregnancy with freedom took back her power over herself. It was life-giving, world-making. Damaris Hill in her own poetic tribute to Assata highlights this drive toward love and community as central to her resistance. In her poem "Truth Is a Mirror in the Hands of God: Assata in 1976," Hill writes:

> For true, from the long end
> of the looking glass, it appears
>
> isolation is one way to quell
> a revolution.[4]

Reflecting on the centrality of community for Black feminist revolutionaries like Assata Shakur and nineteenth-century Creole Voodoo woman Marie Leveau, the poem offers a throughline through history of Black women's refusal to be isolated in their resistance. In many ways, those of us in the Livable Black Futures Project were on our end of the looking glass taking our cues from individuals like Assata to transform our isolation into communal power. For those in our project who had been formally incarcerated, the emergence out of isolation would prove challenging, but thankfully not impossible.

BREAKING THE SILENCE

We sat in silence in the middle of the Pan-African Connection Bookstore in Dallas, Texas, one evening in April 2022. We were surrounded by books, African pottery and garments, and a host of Black-affirming images. I fixated on a large reddish-brown earthen clay pot, thinking about its heaviness and its beauty—imagining what I might plant in it or even what could grow from this gathering. Positioned in a circle, we fumbled over our pasta and pizza, trying to get to know one another. I could tell the storytellers were wondering if they could trust me and the Livable Black Futures Storytelling Project team (D'Andra Willis, Qiana Lewis-Arnold, and Helen Zimba, along with Dr. Allison Tomlinson): if they could trust that what they said to us would matter. We were gathered with formerly incarcerated Black-identified women and for the next phase of our Livable Black Futures Storytelling Project. We were meeting to talk about what it meant to experience gynecological and obstetric medicine while incarcerated. When I think back on it now, that task was already overwhelming. Asking individuals to recall encounters with medicine while imprisoned meant their reaching back into what were painful experiences that triggered other memories as well. Our social worker, Allison, was on hand to support, but it was clear that we were not fully prepared for what was to come.

The prison is a site of foreclosed life, a system embedded in the continuum of stolen Black life, designed to be hidden from view, unlocatable in our consciousness. Slavery "possesses" the prison and its neoliberal logics, as Stephen Dillon contends.[5] Just as slavery possesses the neoliberal carceral state, it too possesses reproduction. Alys Weinbaum identifies what she terms the "slave episteme," the afterlife of a thought system that renders human reproduction's devaluation and extraction as conceivable and that if left unchecked will continue.[6] The logics of the slave episteme are most viscerally felt when we join reproduction with incarceration. The prison cannot sustain life, and thus giving birth in prison is often akin to giving birth to death and loss. People *do* give birth in prison, and they experience gynecological medicine while imprisoned; however, their stories are rarely included in the mainstream discourse on birth justice and reproductive justice. With notable exceptions, such as the work being done by the Prison Policy Initiative,[7] data on birth outcomes, maternal mortality, and infant mortality is often obscured from view. These individuals are perhaps the most affected by intersectional invisibility[8] in reproductive justice research and discourse—where those who are Black, gender expansive, disabled, incarcerated, and economically underresourced (often simultaneously) are often underexamined.

There is a tendency to elevate those who are considered undeserving victims of the crisis of Black maternal health—those who shouldn't die. While celebrity advocates[9] bring attention to the issues affecting Black birthing people, their plights are often overemphasized in contrast to the near dismissal of the circumstances of groups like incarcerated birthing people. Prison abolitionist Mariame Kaba asserts that there are no perfect victims. She reminds us that victims of systemic, often socially sanctioned, violence should not have the truths of their lives flattened in the service of perfect-victim narratives.[10] This chapter raises up the full subjectivities of Black birthing people who have experienced incarceration. It is an account of my engagement with this community in Dallas via our storytelling project. I place their stories in conversation with the more public accounts of Assata Shakur and her political autobiography, *Assata*, as well as the visual artistry of Mary Enoch Elizabeth Baxter (aka Isis Tha Savior) and her account of giving birth while imprisoned. Collectively, these stories offer a narrative and visual dimension to the inhumane treatment of Black birthing people in prison, including shackling of prisoners while they are giving birth, poor medical care, and immediate child separation—thereby producing rippling traumatic effects. Their stories are critical because every modern-day indignity that comes from the denial of reproductive autonomy can be found in incarcerated women's lives.[11]

Only two of our interested storytellers were able to make it to our first in-person meeting, although our initial Zoom recruitment meeting garnered fifteen interested storytellers. This turnout was worrying because we wanted to be able to reach as many individuals as possible and couldn't understand the disparity between the enthusiastic online interest and the actual in-person engagement. Afiya Center executive director Marsha Jones reassured us that the numbers were not a concern. We should do this work to reach whomever we could and keep trying. It was another reminder on why research on underrepresented populations has to be thought differently. Building participation and capacity on research topics that engage marginalized populations takes an incredible amount of labor and time. These realities require an adjustment of traditional standards (such as sample size). Because we had additional meetings scheduled, we were not fully deterred. We just knew that we would have to adjust and do more work to engage with our storytellers. Although our goal was to hold in-person meetings to harness the power of physicality in shared space, we didn't fully anticipate the barriers before our storytellers. They contended with transportation issues, evening work commitments, strict curfew hours for shelters, and more. Their postincarceration lives were full of uncertainty as well as restrictions on their freedom.

We pressed on because we wanted to break the silence around carceral gynecological and obstetric medicine in our immediate communities. Following Dorothy Roberts's assertion that "theories of reproductive freedom must start with the lives of the women at the bottom, not at the top,"[12] we knew that this group was key to our project of reimagining care. Also, scholars such as Crystal Hayes, Carolyn Sufrin, and Jamila Perritt in their article "Reproductive Justice Disrupted: Mass Incarceration as a Driver of Reproductive Oppression" make the case that "mass incarceration, by its very nature, compromises and undermines bodily autonomy and the capacity for incarcerated people to make decisions about their reproductive wellbeing and bodies; this is done through institutionalized racism and is disproportionately done to the bodies of women of color. This violates the most basic tenets of reproductive justice."[13] The struggles of incarcerated birthing people must be ground zero for our battle against reproductive oppression. These issues are intertwined and became more urgent to us as we continued our work.

The silence of the room early on and the reticence to share made sense to me. Here I was twelve years out from my traumatic birthing experiences and I was just now finding language to express what I had been through. Not only is it difficult to find language to express trauma, but society often punishes the vocalizing of unspeakable experience. Shame still functions as a powerful instrument of social control. So there were many factors at play in the silence. Many of us on the research team were also guarded because we were still carrying trauma. One word that constantly circulated among us was *heaviness*—the unbearable weight of these experiences and their attendant traumas. One of our storytellers told us that when you are released from incarceration there is no mental health care transition to process all that you have seen and experienced. You are sent back out into the world with little support beyond limited resources that people share with you. Your survival after incarceration often depends on what resources people are willing to share and tell you about. Interestingly, the organization REBUILD[14] offers a free service helping formerly incarcerated people of color find therapists of color to support them after incarceration. Yet our storytellers were unaware that a program like this existed. Many of them stated that our storytelling work was the first time they had talked in community or with support from others whom they identified with about their experiences. We were surprised to hear this and became even more intentional about producing a safe and judgment-free space.

We tapped into our own experiences supporting incarcerated loved ones. For many of us these issues are close to home when it comes to our proximity to the penal system. The Afiya Center employs formerly incarcerated people. Many of us have relatives who have experienced incarceration or have had negative interactions with law enforcement. As I was thinking about these women, I couldn't help but think about my own grandmother, Lillie Pearl, who experienced incarceration after being convicted of manslaughter during a violent altercation with a male visitor to her home. She was in Parchman Prison in Mississippi—a former plantation and now a center of mass incarceration. When I was born, she had to be escorted to the hospital by prison guards, shackled. Thankfully, her stay ended by the time I was approximately four years old, so I got to grow up with her. For a while, her imprisonment was something we (her grandchildren) spoke about in hushed tones. Sometimes one of us would be bold enough to ask how it had been. She would tell us bits and pieces, largely reciting her survival strategies. One thing I always remembered about her after her incarceration was how she slept on her back with her arms folded, getting extremely startled when awakened from her sleep (often with fear and heavy breathing). The grandchildren would giggle at this, but I think on it now and wonder just how much of those sleeping and waking practices were informed by trauma—all that she had seen. Her silence was also driven by a sense of unworthiness. She had a sweet but self-deprecating way of speaking about herself, often refusing the compliments she so richly deserved. As a child, I often took it as my mission to tell her how great she was. She never really believed me. In fact, she often told me the story about when she was finally released from prison and saw her grandchildren for the first time as a free woman. She said she approached us and I immediately said, "Grandma, you look beautiful!" but one of my other cousins interrupted and said, "Grandma, you look horrible!" She told me that from that interaction she knew she couldn't trust me to tell the truth about how she looked. She would say this jokingly, but part of me believes she was more willing to believe the negative remark because she *felt* horrible. She had experienced the most horrible thing one could experience. The worst yet—as Ella from Toni Morrison's *Beloved* would say. Like those formerly enslaved women trying to shed the horrors of enslavement, I think about my grandmother figuring out how to be after imprisonment. But even as a child, I think I was trying to make my grandmother feel that she was more than what she had experienced: that it was okay, and that she was beautiful just because. I have since lost her, but I was thinking about her when I engaged with these women, all probably navigating similar feelings of shame, unworthiness, trauma, and fear. I took my time engaging them, not knowing when a breakthrough would occur but trusting that it would.

In order to make progress in getting our storytellers to feel safe expressing their views, we also had to construct a setting that was premised on transformative justice. Transformative justice seeks safety and accountability without relying on alienation, punishment, or violence.[15] Part of our challenge was getting our storytellers to trust that we were committed to ending the stigma of incarceration in our work. We did not know it at the time, but reentry had been a bruising process for many of them. In speaking about the difficulty of reentry in a later session, one storyteller stated, "They [those in society] expect you to suffer forever. They want to see your remorse. They don't want you to prosper." It was clear that the shadow of incarceration hung over their lives. Many of them were even in the process of being stripped of their parental rights. Andrea Freeman highlights the historical and progressive efforts to "unmother" black women—to challenge their legitimacy as mothers and stereotype them as "Bad Black mothers."[16] For our storytellers, it was clear that they were fighting to reclaim their identities and move on from the stigma of being incarcerated.[17]

Eventually, in our first session, one of our storytellers, Shani, did share that she was interested in this gathering because she was working to reconnect with her soon-to-be five-year-old son that she had been separated from since his birth. She spoke fondly of him and her hopes to regain custody of him. She also shared some of her background story and said she was a transplant to Texas from Ohio. She often spoke in a hopeful and upbeat tone, espousing statements of "personal responsibility." It made me think of ways the parole system and other agencies often require that formerly incarcerated folks prove that they are reformed. It was clear to me that she could only go so far in telling her story.

Perhaps the biggest beneficiary of our storytellers' reticence was the carceral system. This system relies on the silence of incarcerated people because it keeps them from resisting. DaMaris Hill declares, "A bound woman is a dangerous thing."[18] The question that informs the creation of her book is salient: "What is so threatening about a Black woman bound to her own freedom, one who is also committed to the liberation of others?"[19] Hill's work is a meditation on all the ways Black women have resisted captivity and isolation. I pondered what Hill's words might mean for us in this moment. How could we pierce through the walls that existed between us—not of our own making but created by these carceral traumas? How could we confront the devastating effects of isolation to give voice to unspeakable experiences? How could we build power together?

BREAKING FREE

As I contemplated how to support our storytellers, how to wade through the silence, and how to be prepared for when they were ready or felt safe enough to speak, I returned to Assata Shakur's *Assata*. In addition to being a central text on Black liberation, the work is an indictment of carceral medicine. Assata's birth story informs so much of my understanding of what it means to experience pregnancy as an incarcerated birthing person. Assata was overjoyed to learn that she was pregnant; however, her excitement was met by uncaring prison medical staff. One prison doctor who examined her after an episode of vaginal bleeding dryly informed her that there was a chance she would abort and strongly advised abortion (to complete the process). To this, she responded forcefully, "I don't want no abortion."[20] She writes, "As far as i [sic] could see, they were out to kill my baby. I couldn't lose this baby now, not now. It was meant to be; this baby was our hope. Our hope for the future. I tried to calm myself."[21] Assata's experience reminds us of why it is important to lift up the full framework of reproductive justice, which centers on the right to have children. So many women experiencing incarceration are met with a complete disregard for their pregnancies and their maternal and mental health.

Assata presents a litany of inhumane treatment and medical harm that Shakur and those incarcerated alongside her experienced in prison: both overt violence and passive violence (or the willingness to watch imprisoned folks languish in poor health conditions that often hasten their death). Shakur details how medical conditions at one prison were so bad, the women organized for better health care. As she describes her time in Manhattan Correctional Center (a federal prison), "The health situation was horrible. Women came in off the street and were given no physical exams, no tests, no nothing. They had trouble seeing gynecologists and having their most basic needs met, medical or otherwise."[22] She describes one woman, Charlene (also known as Charlie), who was key in the organizing efforts that she and her fellow inmates engaged in to advocate for better conditions. She was reimprisoned because of a parole violation on a technicality and had to pass the GED to get out of prison. Her spirit was so broken, she didn't have the motivation to study. The only thing that inspired her was the struggle to improve medical care at the correctional center. She led the others in writing complaints to the warden and agitating for someone to address these conditions. Ironically, Charlene ultimately died from an undiagnosed and untreated cancer of the uterus. These were the realities of inmates (or those incarcerated).

The holistic lack of medical care in prisons was felt most deeply by Shakur during her pregnancy with Kakuya. In addition to encouraging her to abort, the prison doctors refused to provide her with key prenatal support, even though she experienced multiple pregnancy complications including bleeding and monilia, a condition of vaginal discharge that chapped her skin so much she could barely walk. More significant is that while she was pregnant, she was unknowingly placed in a cell with a woman who had active tuberculosis. This condition requires the individual to be kept in isolation, yet she spent days in close proximity to Shakur—a contact that threatened her life and that of her unborn child. The prison doctors did everything they could to thwart the outside care Shakur had successfully petitioned to receive. Realizing that she was not going to have access to sufficient prenatal care from prison doctors, she was able to obtain her own doctor, Dr. Ernest Wyman Garrett, who worked to ensure humane treatment for her. In spite of his recommendations, the prison medical staff often refused to comply. She was denied key nutrients like milk and was served pork that they knew she could not eat (which put her in a condition of slow starvation). Prison authorities also required that whenever Dr. Garrett saw her, their own doctor had to be present. This resulted in limiting the number of medical visits Shakur could have because the prison doctor would conveniently not be able to make basic wellness checkups.

In spite of the numerous attempts to harm her during her pregnancy, the state did not prevail, and Shakur was able to give birth with dignity and not be shackled to her bed. Dr. Garrett successfully fought against her shackling during delivery, citing the medical guidance that confirmed the harm of this practice. In the early stages of labor, Shakur had to fight to allow Dr. Garrett to deliver her baby. She had declared that she would deliver the baby by herself rather than allow the prison doctor to do so. She ultimately had a peaceful birth out of the sight of prison surveillance. She also declared, "It's very important for a woman to go through the birth experience with people she trusts."[23] Yet this basic decency of care is often denied incarcerated birthing people, many of whom receive little to no prenatal care and give birth while shackled and surveilled by prison guards.

Shakur's uncharacteristically supportive treatment during delivery ended soon after she gave birth to Kakuya. Dr. Garrett had issued a prescription for Shakur to breastfeed. She was able to do so for one day before they abruptly transported her back to Rikers Island infirmary for any other postnatal care, thereby separating her from her child. When she refused examination, she was beaten by guards and dragged by chains, with only one nurse intervening for them to stop. This occurred within days of delivering her daughter and being separated from her with no notice. The sum of all these indignities is overwhelming to contemplate, and this was even with her having access to her own doctor. The prison staff openly refused to provide her with care, which violated basic medical guidance. They subjected her to physical and mental violence that fully demonstrated the disregard for her life and her role as a mother. Shakur notes that one of the saddest rules she saw while incarcerated occurred in the Middlesex County Workhouse, where children were prohibited from visiting their mothers in jail. She writes, "I could see the children waiting outside, looking up at that ugly old building with sad, frustrated faces. Their mothers would run to the window that faced the parking lot just to get a glimpse of their children. Yelling out of the window was a no-no, but once in a while somebody would get carried away. Sometimes their frantic screams went unheard."[24] The frantic screams of the mothers highlight scenes of despair that affected both mothers and children. They can also be read in the historical context of slavery and the ongoing assault on Black motherhood after slavery. These realities call up how Black women writers have harnessed the rhetorical power of what Joanne Braxton calls the "outraged mother" to critique and condemn racial injustice as early as the slave era and continuing well beyond it. Braxton explains that the outraged mother "travels alone through the darkness to impart a sense of identity and 'belongingness' to her child. She sacrifices and improvises to create the vehicles necessary for the survival of the flesh and spirit. Implied in all her actions and fueling her heroic ones is abuse of her people and her person."[25] The outraged mother speaks on behalf of her people as well as herself, and her rhetorical force expresses the value of both. In this sense, Assata Shakur is a quintessential outraged mother naming all the ways her ability to mother her child was foreclosed by the state and highlighting the intentional practices of the state to sever the mother-child bonds of those incarcerated.

In recounting her experience as a mother whose maternal agency and authority were denied by the state and in lifting up the experiences of so many mothers who have experienced the same, Shakur highlights how prisons are full of outraged mothers. Much as in slavery times, these mothers have been denied their own right to parent. It is important to call attention to the fact that the desire to sustain Black life in a fundamentally anti-Black society holds tremendous contradiction. Joy James describes those caught up in these conflicting stances "Captive Maternals": "those most vulnerable to violence, war, poverty, police, and captivity; those whose very existence enables the possessive empire that claims and dispossesses them."[26] Figures like Assata Shakur exist within what James calls a "Black Matrix," a fulcrum that functions when captives leverage their power. She asserts that theorizing through the fulcrum can enable liberation because "the deliberative faculties shared among the least recognized, shaped by battle, offer new theories as leverage for freedom."[27] It is through this lens that I read the power of Shakur's words that end her poem "Love": "We are pregnant with freedom / We are a conspiracy." It is a theory that serves as leverage for freedom. It announces that the genocidal intentions of the prison will not prevail and that life can be lived against a compelled service to the state and even as a disruption to it.

ABOLITION MEDICINE

More than a personal narrative of indignities she experienced in seeking medical treatment and attending to her child (as well as similar denials experienced by her fellow inmates), Assata's experience evinces the need for *abolition medicine*.[28] Abolition medicine is an outgrowth of the public discourse on prison abolition (a social movement and a visionary framework), most notably spearheaded by activist Mariame Kaba (following the paths made by revolutionary thinkers such as Angela Davis and Ruth Wilson Gilmore), who names abolition as a process of building a society that would make prisons and police obsolete. Although abolition's detractors dismiss this work as merely destructive, abolition is not about destroying but about building something new, with the understanding that some systems simply cannot be reformed—they must be remade. Kaba asserts that "policing and incarceration have always been grounded in anti-Blackness, Native erasure, and protection of property."[29] Given that foundation, abolition demands that we divest from these harmful systems and create the world in which we want to live.[30] Abolition is grounded in principles of cooperation rather than individualism, mutual aid rather than self-preservation. It is an effort to move our society to embrace a different vision of safety and justice.

This vision of safety and justice also needs to be enacted in the medical space, which is bound up in carceral logics. There is a need to decarcerate medicine on many levels. Doctors Nhi

Tran, Aminta Kouyate, and Monica U. Hahn make the point that "US health care intertwines with the US carceral state when clinicians use their authority and power to reinforce patterns of racial oppression."[31] Throughout the history of medicine, we see carceral logics shaping conditions of care: inequitable toxicology screening in Black mothers and newborns, a disregard for the pain of Black patients, and the use of "nonadherence"/noncompliance justifications to employ punitive measures against patients who have complex needs/circumstances affecting their ability to align with recommended treatment plans, for example. Even in the jargon of medical science, we see terms like *incarcerated gravid uterus*, which describes the process that occurs when a retroverted uterus does not resolve beyond mid-gestation and the uterine corpus becomes confined in the hollow of the sacrum, resulting in a displaced cervix.[32] (See also other terms like *incarcerated hernia* and *incarcerated procidentia*.) What these terms demonstrate is that judgment and bias infuse medical jargon. That which is "incarcerated" is noncompliant, stuck in a place where it should not be or misplaced. Trapped. Unruly. Much like the ableist judgment inherent in the term *incompetent cervix*, logics of bias permeate medical discourse itself. They also reveal how medical care often ascribes innocence and guilt to patients and their bodies in ways that also implicitly affect who is deserving of care and compassion. The lack of compassion in the terminology signals this. Esther Kaner writes that health care is also undergirded by forms of control and "hegemonic configurations of health [that] encourage conformity and compliance."[33] It reinforces patient docility and punishes any forms of resistance, and Black people are usually caught in the difficult situation of working to advocate for themselves in a system that has historically disregarded and exploited them. That system, instead of acknowledging these contexts, often deems black people as "unruly," especially if they are economically underresourced. Khiara Bridges makes the point that "women's bodies *behave* as unruly when they are constantly measured, quantified, weighed, gauged, or otherwise assessed within a technology that speaks in terms of normal and abnormal. Variations from the norm become anxiety-marked occasions for further surveillance and the possibility of disciplining the body back to normality."[34] When we consider incarcerated patients in this context, they are always already unruly, noncompliant, and nonadherent. This is deeply reflected in the lack of care extended to them.

Correspondingly, when we consider what it looks like to enact abolition medicine, we need to embrace a different vision of health care and notions of care more broadly. The "care" in health care has been so fraught with problems and contradictions that some exclusively refer to the health care system as the medical-industrial complex in order to draw attention to the dehumanizing, depersonalized, profit-centered enterprise of medicine.[35] What would it look like if our medical systems were instead grounded in equity, patient-centered autonomy, and self-determination?[36] What would it mean for our health care system to take seriously the "moral, ethical, and professional obligation to use its social powers to interrogate and disrupt systems with a history of harming people"?[37] These questions are at the heart of the critical work of abolition medicine because it requires us to envision a new set of possibilities not inherent in the structures in which we function. It requires stepping outside of ingrained practices and undoing the ones that are responsible for causing harm. Esther Kaner offers some prescriptions: challenging the tendency to frame patient behaviors through the lens of criminality; refraining from accusing patients of malingering; increasing empathy;

resisting the urge to chastise patients for things like weight and nonadherence to treatment regimens and instead seeing patients as dealing with complex factors that affect their choices; and committing to dismantling the oppressive structures that make many of us ill in the first place.[38] What Kaner describes here can also be named as reproductive justice. Abolition medicine and reproductive justice are deeply intertwined and are inherently invested in the same objectives.

This is also why any understanding of abolition medicine and reproductive justice has to begin with incarcerated patients. Although carceral logics certainly permeate the medical space beyond the prison, the harm of these logics is exacerbated in prison, where feelings of undeservingness of care and patient blame permeate the space. Carceral health care is a site of concentrated injustice that is a microcosm for the medical harms that exist beyond the prison. These harmful logics are not only intertwined but instructive for how we might truly achieve reproductive justice.

THE BOX

Although Assata Shakur's story demonstrates poor conditions of medical care for those who are incarcerated, we don't have much insight into experiences of incarcerated birthing people.[39] Their health outcomes are often disaggregated from data on maternal mortality. In fact, the Centers for Disease Control's 2022 report on maternal mortality during the onset of the Covid-19 pandemic does not specify if incarcerated birthing people were included in the numbers.[40] Rarely does data on incarcerated birthing people get centered in broader reports on maternal health. They are perpetually boxed in, closed off, contained away from others. Having to check boxes on applications that ask if they have been incarcerated, they know that checking the box can imperil their efforts. This is what our formerly incarcerated storytellers contended with. How could they escape the boxes in which they had been placed, and how could they move forward? In our second meeting, we focused on these boxes and had our storytellers interrogate them with the help of a local creative writer, scholar, and Black birthing person, Dr. Angela Mack. As we embarked on the exercise, I felt an intangible sense of opening—hoping that confronting these boxes would give us language to put to the trauma.

I'm Takin' My Freedom

At the top of our second meeting, which we held virtually to mitigate barriers to participation, Angela had requested to have Jill Scott's "Golden" playing. We wanted to foreground the notion of freedom because we had an overwhelming sense that our storytellers still felt unfree. As "Golden" boomed through the Zoom space, we all bounced to the music smiling and welcoming the storytellers in. I was overjoyed to see the Zoom space begin to fill with people, as little boxes popped up on my screen, continuing to expand the space. Because we had switched to virtual, more of them were able to participate. We had grown from two to ten. It was in this moment that I felt thankful for the virtual space even more. While we wanted to be in close community through physicality, this was not possible for this group without great effort and uneven results. Although Covid-19 has been a tragic era for our world, it did force institutions and industries to think through notions of access more critically. And these pathways made it possible for our storytellers to engage in experiences that they otherwise would have been cut off from because of issues of transportation and work schedules. They were at various sites—at home, at work, in their cars, but they were here in shared space and community. I felt a sense of promise just by having more of them make the time to show up.

Angela opened with her own poem "My Name, My Freedom Poem," which set the tone in an even deeper way. We listened as she read:

> My Name
> is not some statistic tatted on me
> as a Black woman burdened with the blues
>
> My name
> is not obesity, preeclampsia, or neglect
> I am not some subset
> of some medical doctor's experiment
>
> My name is not
> my mama's history, nor my dad's
> it's not the bloodiness of an unruly womb
>
> My name
> is not stacks of risk factors and potential complications
> it's not a death sentence to a maternal tomb
>
> My name
> is not erasure, being ignored, being unheard, or overruled
> it's not the lack of quality care or from pain that's not assumed
>
> My name
> is not my disfigured breasts, my scarred lungs, or having a
>   Cesarean birth
> it's not what others make conclusions from
> but my Name is my value and my worth
>
> My name
> is bearing witness to my body in the ways she breaks all the rules
> she speaks life to those who don't want my living
> she is my ancestors' greatest tool

My name
is Here, Now, Present, and Being
My name is Angela, and it's in me that my Future is Breathing

Angela's poem lays bare the experiences of far too many Black birthing people—objectified as unruly bodies because of their various health conditions, their weight, their Blackness. Like *Assata*'s litany of medical harm experienced by Shakur and her fellow inmates, "My Name" sets out a litany of abuses and harms that Angela, as the speaker, has experienced. I think of Audre Lorde's poem "A Litany for Survival," which echoes the devastating refrain, "We were never meant to survive."[41] Lorde's intellection speaks for those of us who live just on the edge of foreclosure, just on the edge of defeat, but are endeavoring to live beyond fear. Angela's words respond to histories of medical trauma (personal and collective) to assert her humanity and the humanity of those unnamed in the archives. She is naming the pain and naming herself in the process. In describing herself, she is refusing the narrative that the medical system might write for her. As a woman of size, Angela has faced various forms of carceral medical treatment, from the surveillance of her body to doctors' tendency to judge and blame her and her weight for her medical ailments. She vulnerably shared her experience with the storytellers, and her story palpably resonated with the others as they thought on how they had been named and defined by systems designed to keep them in a state of unfreedom.

Angela then gave the storytellers a prompt to draw a box on a sheet of paper and place into this drawing the various harms they had experienced, with the goal of naming, containing, and eventually freeing themselves from them. As we played music, the storytellers went off camera and wrote. When everyone returned, they were ready to share thoughts drawn from deep contemplation. Rather than get right into the sharing of the difficult experiences they had placed in their boxes, Angela queried them on what a box meant to them. Responses included words like *isolation, barriers, closed off,* and even *a comfort zone.* One storyteller lamented that since reentering society after incarceration she still felt confined to a box. What the storytellers revealed was that even as they worked to move forward from their pasts, they were still being placed in boxes and experiencing barriers and isolation.

Slowly, storytellers shared what they had put in their boxes. One predominant narrative was experiences of physical and sexual abuse even before entering prison. The water began to break. Storytellers told stories of forced abortions, sexual assault, child abuse, and unfortunately generational abuse experienced by elders and passed down to children. In this moment, the abuse-to-prison pipeline was made plain for me. The storytellers had in common not only having been incarcerated but also having experienced some form of physical and/or sexual abuse, along with those they loved. Studies such as *The Sexual Abuse to Prison Pipeline*[42] show how girls who have been physically and sexually abused are criminalized in ways similar to those described for the school-to-prison pipeline. As the storytellers told stories of their boxes, it became apparent how they were victims of the criminalization of being abused, being poor, or being mentally ill.

As we unpacked what was in our boxes, storytellers were encouraged to get control over them by closing them and thinking about how they could reframe themselves. Angela reentered the conversation and asked the storytellers to take a new page, draw a picture frame, and place words of affirmation for themselves about how they saw themselves versus the negative societal narrative. Responses began flowing: "beautiful, God's child, strong, worthy, independent, successful, determined, survivor . . ." Our time was coming to an end, but we were only just beginning to unpack the stories. Although our focus for the study was experiences with carceral medicine, it was clear that many factors had compounded to result in the storytellers' imprisonment and their treatment while they were incarcerated. We had begun the process, but it was clear that we had only touched the surface. The storytellers were not yet ready to close their boxes.

We Demand Dignity

Following the powerful session with Angela Mack, we reassembled on Zoom the next week. The heaviness of our waterbreaking was still in the air. As we welcomed storytellers into the space, I could tell that we still needed to deepen our conversation. We had facilitated an opening up of the storytellers about their histories and the experiences that had shaped them, but we weren't quite there to engage their experiences while incarcerated. My research partners and I had also agreed that perhaps a more targeted set of questions could help us go further into their experience with gynecological medicine while incarcerated. Once we completed our ritual grounding practice, we posed this question at the top of the meeting: *"You have unique knowledge because of your experience with medicine while incarcerated (especially with regard to your sexual and reproductive health). Did you receive care or not? If not, what would you have liked to receive?"*

We played music as they journaled, and when it was time to share, our first response was telling. One storyteller, Blue, deadpanned, "They don't give you any health care." Immediately, I saw heads nodding in their Zoom boxes, people typing into the chat,

"That's right," as I processed all that that single sentence meant. What it confirmed for me was the necropolitical underpinnings of the carceral system. Achille Mbembé theorizes necropolitics as a political calculus, growing out of legacies of colonialism and slavery, for who lives and who dies, whose life is valuable and whose life is expendable.[43] The penal system sees inmates as disposable, as objects to be exploited, managed, and contained. Soon their responses began to resemble Angela's litany of harm, with many storytellers recounting horrific experiences they had had while incarcerated. One shared that she had witnessed someone die from an untreated asthma attack. Another described the indignity of random strip searches where sanitary napkins had to be removed in front of others. Much as Assata Shakur recounted being housed with someone with active tuberculosis, many storytellers recalled exposure to staph infections, scabies, and other contagious illnesses. We know that Covid-19 has been especially devastating for those incarcerated. The Equal Justice Initiative reports that incarcerated people are infected with Covid-19 at a rate five times higher than the nonincarcerated population.[44] There is also a great deal of underreporting because inmates are rarely tested for Covid. If this recent fact is an indicator, then what the storytellers recalled confirms the systemic medical neglect of those incarcerated.

Of course, the central experiences of our storytellers focused on pregnancy and childbirth. A storyteller noted that her sister had been pregnant in prison and had received little to no medical care. "You just stay pregnant. You do not go and see a nurse or anything until it's time for delivery and then they take that baby right from you."[45] This story also reflected Assata Shakur's abrupt separation from her daughter and the lack of care for her postpartum health. Another storyteller recalled how a fellow inmate who was four months pregnant had been taken to a hospital off premises and had returned after losing her child through what inmates suspected was a forced abortion.[46] A similarly difficult story came from a storyteller who dealt with seizures and mental illness and had had a miscarriage in prison. She had been unaware that she was carrying a child, and she repeated to our group, "I had a whole baby in me. I lost a whole baby not knowing I was pregnant." A whole baby. I linger on her words. The baby was whole and growing inside of her and she did not know. I think also about the homonyms *whole* and *hole*. As this storyteller's words reverberated in the space, it seemed that her loss had left a hole, yet to be filled, a loss for which mourning was still ongoing.

These accounts reflect works like the visual art triptych "Ain't I a Woman," by Mary Enoch Elizabeth Baxter (aka Isis Tha Savior).[47] Constructed as a story in three acts, the video moves us through her arrest, her pregnancy and delivery, and her public advocacy once she is released. It takes us through a series of searing images of her harrowing experience giving birth, from being shackled to the bed for forty-three hours, to being treated with psychotropic drugs because of her trauma, to her separation from her child. Making connections to her experience and the experiences of Black mothers in the transatlantic slave trade, she raps, "The flashback screams echo from a slave ship, wreckage, a hard lesson, but tell me what's the deeper message." Isis Tha Savior places her experience within the context of chattel slavery, drawing an even deeper illustration of the dehumanization of incarceration. She then goes on to describe the isolation she experienced while giving birth—having no visitors and not getting to nurse her son. The imagery of the film is haunting. Isis is pictured in a cavernous space in her orange jumpsuit being shackled to the bed by often faceless, emotionless medical staff as she cries out for help and pleads to be unshackled.[48] The film also depicts various kinds of carceral geographies (public housing, public schools, and under-resourced neighborhoods), all of which place a stranglehold on the life possibilities for Black people.

Amid all of this, though, we see how Isis Tha Savior, like Assata Shakur, refuses to have her life foreclosed because she is in prison. Nicole Fleetwood offers, "While Baxter's video provides a vivid account of the carceral continuum, it also sets up an important tension that many artists in this study [*Marking Time*] have described: that art-making in prison serves as acts of freedom that cannot be completely governed by prison regulation—and yet these articulations of freedom dreams, to borrow a phrase from Robin D.G. Kelley, remain bounded by the very institution that holds them as captives."[49] What Fleetwood describes is similar to the idea of the Captive Maternal. In the necropolitical context of the prison and the broader society, which has been shaped by anti-Blackness, assertions of one's agency and viability are bound to the system even as they sustain the structures that create the oppressive conditions of their lives. I also read Baxter's work alongside the conversations of our incarcerated storytellers, who bravely shared and opened up to strangers what was often unspeakable injustice they had witnessed or even experienced firsthand. In one section of the video is the line "Restore dignity to incarcerated women." I deeply felt this directive as I worked with the storytellers to grapple with all the ways their dignity had been disregarded while they were incarcerated. Near the end of our time, one storyteller asked, almost in desperation, "How do you get past the trauma? Do you ever recover?" We began to share the mental health resources that we had gathered to support them, and our social worker Allison chimed in; however, all of us knew that the systems that structure the carceral continuum and the abuse-to-prison pipeline as well as health care systems remain. We ended our meeting with a sense of release but also unsure of how to move forward. We engaged in a grounding practice before we ended by playing Jhene Aiko's "Trigger Protection Mantra." As Aiko's voice faded, I quietly prayed for their protection and mine.

TRAUMA AND TIME THEFT

Joy James describes all the ways time is stolen from those who are captive: the time of captivity does not recognize childhood or motherhood; lives and livelihoods are shortened by poor health care; Black defendants are given longer sentences than their white counterparts for similar offenses; they lose leisure and the time it takes to recover from fatigue and violence, and so on.[50] As we entered our last meeting, we were all feeling the crush of time (we needed more time together, but time was running out). After that last meeting, my mind was filled with concerns. I thought about the forward progression of time and how it moves so slowly for those incarcerated and then speeds up when they are released. They have to contend with lost time and time passing them by. It was May 6, the Friday before Mother's Day. We were prepared to make this last meeting a precelebration for them, but as we were planning, there was a leaked Supreme Court opinion by Justice Samuel Alito that portended the fall of *Roe v. Wade*. The case, *Dobbs v. Jackson Women's Health Organization*,[51] basically proposed stripping the right to abortion nationwide and placing the issue squarely in the states' hands. In Texas, we knew that this decision meant the end of legal abortion in the state. My co-researchers showed up to the Zoom exhausted, having been busy strategizing and planning actions in response to this moment that we had all known was coming. The leaked document added proof to that. It was all so much to contend with.

I thought about our storytellers, working so hard to reenter society and live freely. I knew this must be triggering for them to have another dimension of their lives criminalized. We know that the criminalization of abortion bears most heavily on Black and Brown women because they are often targets of the carceral state. What did it mean for them to hold this news?

For this last meeting, our goal was to focus on where we could go from here and what we could do with the stories we had been given. The storytellers agreed that people needed to know what medical treatment was like for incarcerated women, especially in relation to their gynecological and obstetric health. I wrote in my notes the need to do more amplifying of available statistical data on pregnancy outcomes for incarcerated women as well as various kinds of challenges that incarcerated women face in receiving medical care. I was thinking of the medical inhumanity evidenced in their stories. As the field of medical humanities grows, it is important to interrogate the "humanity" that is implied. Humanities as a field is concerned with the human condition. The experiences of incarcerated subjects require that we account for the inhumane acts enacted on vulnerable people. What descriptors do we need so as not to obscure how medical experience varies widely depending on one's social status?

Another thing our storytellers advocated for was for everyone to commit to their own wellness in light of all the ways they had been harmed across time. Healing was central.

One storyteller noted, "We absolutely have to do our own healing so that we can advocate and change policy, so that our kids can live and thrive." I found this sentiment both beautiful and overwhelming. The storytellers wanted to heal from the past so that they could enable livable Black futures. This prompted me to think on the title of our storytelling project and what it meant in light of their narratives. It was hard trying to think about futurity given the bleak realities of the clock ticking toward the fall of *Roe v. Wade*. We were running out of time.

Holding this contradiction of the impending fall of *Roe v. Wade* and the desire to envision pathways for Black viability (including the right to give birth with dignity and to raise children in a safe society) to me most centrally highlighted the meaning of reproductive justice. The issue our storytellers were concerned about alongside abortion was how to survive. They wanted to sustain their lives and the lives of their loved ones. It wasn't just about being able to end a pregnancy (or not being subject to forced birth) when the state had shown that it was not invested in their lives and was in some senses actively working to foreclose them. "Black Lives Matter" has become a rallying cry, and in reproductive justice this resonates deeply. The experiences of incarcerated birthing people throw the devaluation of Black lives into sharp relief. There is a complete disregard for life in the carceral state (multiple levels of indignity, disregard, family separation, and on). We cannot realize reproductive justice if we don't center the ongoing assault on this deeply vulnerable collective.

At the end of our last session, Shani, who had spoken up at our first session about not having her five-year-old son, felt moved to open up about how she was feeling ahead of Mother's Day. This Mother's Day would be painful, she admitted, because she was nearing the five-year deadline to have housing and financial stability so that she could get her son out of the state's care and bring him home with her. As she spoke, it became increasingly clear that this was not going to be likely. She noted that old charges had begun resurfacing on her records and she was not being given information about her visitation rights. She lamented, "He's going to be five next month. And I'm still struggling, trying to find a way to keep afloat. And it's like walking on eggshells here in this city [Dallas]." As she spoke, the others related deeply to her pain. Many of them also felt as if they were walking on eggshells trying to live a free life. They knew that one false move could send them back to prison. There was so much at stake. This reality sheds light on the mental dimensions of the harm created by criminalizing abortion. It is just one more means to make birthing people unfree.

These formerly incarcerated individuals are attempting to rewrite the narrative of their lives and claim their names. This is the challenge facing many people marginalized in reproductive justice discourse. Because they are often not the perfect victims (or don't align with those for whom the mainstream public will feel empathy), their stories are often removed from public consciousness when in actuality they should be centered. In our prior session (session 2), our facilitator Angela had encouraged them to spend time meditating on their names and how they could reclaim their names. I knew that for many of them this exercise required more than just one evening. It would be a process because they were trying to reclaim a sense of self after being defined by the state. They were still in search of freedom.

CHAPTER SIX

Policing Black Birth

Affirmation

I claim my right as a Black parent to give birth without state intervention. I fight this fight against a backdrop of histories of attacks on Black motherhood and ongoing structural efforts to separate Black families.

Like the prison system, the family-policing system frays social bonds and strains the ability of community members to resist oppression and organize politically. In our protests against anti-Black state violence, we should amplify the voices of parents who fight every day for their families in the halls of family court and in their communities.

—Dorothy Roberts, *Torn Apart*

In listening to the stories of the formerly incarcerated storytellers we communed with, I was struck by the ways their stories overlapped with those of our first group of Black birthing people, who had not experienced incarceration but had experienced policing of their birth experiences. The issue of carcerality (acts of surveillance and criminalization in particular) ran throughout our conversations. In so many ways, the criminalization of Black people is very apparent during delivery and postpartum. Our storytellers reported being hypersurveilled and monitored in ways that made them feel like they were under suspicion. Many of them had been separated from their children at some point in their lives. For many of them, their experiences with family policing had begun in the delivery room. One formerly incarcerated storyteller, Shani, made clear to us the long-term impact of policing Black birth because she was still living the effects of state intervention into her life and pregnancy. At the end of our experience, she released a lot of what she had been holding with regard to her separation from her child. She was struggling with the emotional pain of not being able to reunite with her now five-year-old son, who had been born just before she was incarcerated. Her story poured out like waterbreaking as she shared her complex journey. In addition to wanting to participate in our storytelling research to offer insight into her experience of gynecological and obstetric medicine while incarcerated, she wanted to share a current indignity she was experiencing in the aftermath. She said, "I am here because I wanted someone to know what happened to my son. He is now a part of the system. His adoption was unnecessary because I'm here and capable of taking care of my son."

Shani told her story in a nonlinear way (a sign of ongoing trauma), but it was clear that she had never truly been given a chance to mother her son. She also told her story through labored breathing caused by a worsening respiratory condition. She didn't have access to needed medical care and was relying on Medicaid for her support at the time. Arline Geronimus's theory of weathering is very relevant here. Geronimus argues that Black people experience "early health deterioration because of the cumulative impact of repeated experience with social or economic adversity and political marginalization. On a physiological level, persistent, high-effort coping with acute and chronic stressors can have a profound effect on health."[1] This early health deterioration can be read alongside what Saidiya Hartman describes as the "afterlives of slavery": "skewed life chances, limited access to health and education, premature death, incarceration, and impoverishment."[2] I think about Shani's ongoing stress of not knowing if she would be able to regain custody of her son and how that showed up in her breathing. She wheezed in a clear manifestation of physical pain intertwined with emotional pain. We all worried about her well-being.

When Shani learned she was pregnant, she was experiencing houselessness. Moving between shelters, she was told she had to gather resources for her son quickly enough to be able to keep him in her care. She reached out to some of the same support systems that she had relied on in the lead-up to the birth of her older daughter. However, in this current case, she became a target for surveillance and concern that she was not equipped to care for her unborn child. She solicited churches and charity groups to secure the baby supplies that she was told she needed. During this time, she developed preeclampsia, a condition of high blood pressure that affects Black women at higher rates than any other group and can become deadly. She had to deliver early, resulting in her son being born prematurely. In the hospital, she was visited by child protective services workers who determined not only that she had not secured the necessary supplies in time but also that a homeless shelter was no environment in which she could bring home a baby born prematurely. They pressured her to make arrangements to send her child to a relative, and the child was later placed in state custody. Because of the intervention of the state at the birth of her son, she was denied the dignity of bonding with him. Since that time, she had not been able to regain custody of him. During the separation from her son, Shani endured incarceration and probation. She was told that if she stayed out of jail, she would be able to reunite with her son when he turned five. He was turning five within months of her participation in our storytelling research, and all she could focus on was getting her son back.

Shani is one of the many victims of policing the Black body during the pregnancy and birthing process. Her story brought us into greater realization of the insidious ways that the state surveils and criminalizes Black pregnancy. On hearing Shani's story, I thought back to all the ways our storytellers described feeling policed in the hospital, to the point of having child protective services called on them. They experienced an overwhelming amount of indignity during and after giving birth. This aligns with the excessive drug testing of Black birthing people during delivery as well as the criminalization of home births. I look to Black birth as a site of policing that offers significant insight into the pervasive ways the state sanctions and often separates Black families. Not just the womb itself but the act of giving birth is a criminalized space for Black birthing people, with ruinous consequences. This chapter speaks to both these devastating impacts and our storytellers' resistance to being policed.

UNMOTHERING BLACK WOMEN AND BIRTHING PEOPLE

Birth is a key site for the delegitimization of Black mothering and parenting. For Black parents, births, instead of being beautiful experiences, are often mired in criminalization. This works as a part of a larger systemic effort to "unmother" Black women and birthing people. Andrea Freeman describes the process of unmothering Black women, noting that since slavery, dehumanizing Black mothers (divorcing them from conceptions of good mothering) has been central to the racial project of entrenching political, financial, and social inequality.[3] By placing pregnant Black mothers and birthing people under suspicion, this practice emerges in the medical space in troubling ways. In Texas and during the time of our storytelling project, the issue of suspicion was magnified because Senate Bill 8 (otherwise known as the "Heartbeat Bill") encouraged state residents to conduct their own vigilante surveillance by reporting anyone suspected of having an abortion. These layers of suspicion operate along a continuum of criminalizing Black motherhood that emerges in legislation, surveillance, and the family policing system.

With respect to legislation, the policing of the Black womb is most apparent in the ongoing restrictions on abortion rights and by extension bodily autonomy. Michele Goodwin's work *Policing the Womb* illuminates how "the recent robust lawmaking that restricts when and under what circumstances women may access reproductive healthcare rights functions not only to undermine women's constitutional rights but also leads to the surveillance of their reproduction, criminalization of their conduct during pregnancy, and ultimately the burdening of their health."[4] For Black birthing people, this legislation only exacerbates what they have experienced for many years. The stress that the policing of the womb creates for Black birthing people has an immense negative impact on their health and in many respects the health of the child. Essentially, the overturning of *Roe v. Wade* and the enactment of other measures that encourage the surveillance of pregnant people make a terrible environment in which to be a pregnant Black person even worse.

In addition to Goodwin's exploration of the ways the state imperils Black birthing and Black motherhood, Dorothy Roberts's

Torn Apart provides an overarching critical assessment of the family policing system and its harms to Black and Brown families. She makes the point that "regulating and destroying Black families—in addition to Latinx, Indigenous, and other impoverished families—in the name of child protection has been essential to the 'ongoing white supremacist nation building project' to quote Mariame Kaba, as much as prisons and police. Like the prison system, the family-policing system frays social bonds and strains the ability of community members to resist oppression and organize politically."[5] Taken together, what Goodwin and Roberts describe here is an intensifying assault on pregnant Black people. The hypersurveillance of Black women and birthing people during and after pregnancy initiates the unmothering of Black women and birthing people and the separation of Black families. While Black women and birthing people and their families feel this most intimately, it is clear that childbirth in our present day is becoming more and more criminalized for all wombholders. Roberts characterizes this criminalization of birth and the wholesale attack on all birthing people in the aftermath of *Dobbs v. Jackson* as all-pervasive. In an interview with Dahlia Lithwick, she asserts: "Today we see that there is very clearly an anti-abortion right-wing strategy of reproductive control that includes both the criminalization of people who want to have babies and the criminalization of those seeking abortion." Criminalization expands beyond abortion to "the criminalization of having children; the criminalization of being a mother in a racist white supremacist society that doesn't meet people's needs."[6]

And it is not simply criminalization of Black mothering. It is criminalization of mothering by Black people who are poor, or are contending with mental instability, or seek more autonomy over their birthing processes, or do not align with the heteronormative ideal. How does one challenge this system? My research found people subject to these conditions who were pushing back and fighting against them. In some cases, they were successful in keeping their children, but the real questions for me are, What has been the expense to their well-being? In what ways have these interlocking systems of oppression that produce indignity and harm weathered them? How are these experiences a part of the same dynamics? While the responses to these questions in relation to the stories I explore in this chapter remain to be seen, it is imperative that we factor them into the conversation about the criminalization of pregnancy, birthing, and motherhood. These structures produce collateral damage in families that we are only beginning to uncover.

BIRTHING UNDER THE CRIMINALIZING GAZE

Even before a Black child is born, data show that Black women and birthing people experience more suspicion during the pregnancy and delivery process than their white counterparts in that they are drug tested at higher rates and are more likely to have reports made about them to child protective services. A 2023 report by Frank Edwards et al. in *Health Equity* on the relationship between medical professional reports and child welfare investigations found that "racial inequities in child welfare investigations of infants persist, although the magnitude of inequity varies by state. Per capita rates of investigations of Black infants following medical professionals' reports increased ~230% between 2010 and 2019."[7] Child welfare reports focusing on Black infants by medical professionals in hospital settings are on the rise and represent an extension of the family policing system well before Black parents even take their children home from the hospital. According to Edwards et al., "Medical professional reports are a significant contributor to the stark racial inequities in these child welfare investigations both in general and specifically related to substance use."[8] How can Black women and birthing people trust that they will not have their dignity assaulted when they go to deliver their children?

Alongside Edwards's study, a 2023 study by the University of Pittsburgh Center for Innovative Research in Gender and Health Equity showed similar troubling trends in the drug testing of Black women and birthing people while in the hospital delivering their children. It reported that "hospitals are more likely to give drug tests to Black women delivering babies than white women, regardless of the mother's history of substance use."[9] Concurrently, it found that "Black women were less likely than white women to test positive for drugs."[10] These findings are deeply concerning because they reveal that there is little correlation between the suspicion of drug use by Black mothers and birthing people and the reality. Black women often are viewed through the tropes of Welfare Queen and Crack Addict Mother. Drug testing at childbirth is one of the main ways Black women and birthing people are unmothered during pregnancy and delivery. Moreover, even efforts to address this racial disparity have had limited success. "Some health systems use specific protocols to determine who gets urine testing, including factors like late entry to prenatal care or preterm birth, which disproportionately impact Black women, Sarah Roberts, study author and professor at the University of California San Francisco, wrote in an email to Axios."[11] Roberts added that "protocols based on factors such as these [delayed prenatal care and preterm birth] essentially just institutionalize the racism that exists when providers are left on their own to decide whose urine to test."[12] The subjective nature of decisions on whose urine to test and the protocols that leave room for disparity in how they are applied show the systemic nature of the criminalization and policing of Black women and birthing people in hospitals. There is a need to have deeper conversations on these issues in medical education. Systemic racism still very much infuses medical care, and the need to address the biases that health care systems amplify is critical. Systemic racism has a totalizing effect—so much so that it is as omnipresent as the weather. As Christina Sharpe explains in *In the Wake: On Blackness and Being*, "The weather is the totality of our environments; the weather is the total climate; and that climate is antiblack."[13] Shani was caught in a swirl of conditions infused with anti-Blackness (namely, the state's disregard for Black motherhood and its ongoing practice of separating Black children from their families). Black people have a long-standing and valid distrust of health care spaces (due to historic harms experienced within them),[14] and the additional suspicions of criminality directed at Black women and birthing people only exacerbate their distrust.

One of our storytellers, Laila, voiced this distrust intensely. She had deeply experienced surveillance and the criminalizing gaze when delivering her son—an unexpected pregnancy just before the onset of the Covid-19 pandemic. When she learned she was pregnant, she sought support for an abortion. Senate Bill 8 had not yet taken effect, and she was given what she thought was medication to facilitate her abortion. Months later, she experienced intense pain and went to the hospital to be seen. There she learned that she was still pregnant and in delivery. Naturally, panic set in and she began to voice her distress. Laila did not want children, and the thought of becoming a mother within hours was overwhelming. She processed these feelings out loud in the hospital and in front of the medical staff. As she continued to speak, she noticed a marked shift in how members of the medical staff were treating her, particularly the white nurses, who she felt were silently judging her. She didn't feel safe (especially given that she was already feeling betrayed about the failed abortion, where she suspected that she had never been given abortion medication). She wanted a Black nurse and someone she felt she could trust to help her process what was happening. She told us, "I had an abortion, I thought, but I was actually pregnant. I don't want kids. So I was cussing through the pain, and I felt unsafe." Laila's authentic response to her situation placed her in a precarious and vulnerable position at the hospital. She felt that prior medical staff had deceived her when she had sought an abortion, yet she was now having to trust a new set of medical professionals who were in place to help her deliver an unexpected and unwanted pregnancy.

Pain and shock worked together on Laila's body and mind in ways that made her a target for surveillance. Thankfully, she had a connection to a doula, who traveled to the hospital to be with her once she realized what was happening. The doula's presence mitigated some of the panic, but not before the medical staff began to surreptitiously document her actions and alert child protective services. Rather than comfort her, the medical staff viewed her behavior through the lens of criminality. She sensed that and asked for certain staff not to engage with her. They called a child protective services worker and had them listen over the phone to what was occurring in the room. Laila recalled,

> I was dealing with all this pain and confusion and talking about it through delivery. I didn't know until after the fact that they had a social service worker over the phone listening to what I was saying. Then after the birth she comes in to talk me pretending like she wants to talk about breastfeeding. They started asking me all these questions about the father. They were planning to take my baby from me.

The level of violation here is significant. In the process of facilitating her birth, medical staff were also poised to report Laila to child protective services and were recording her without her consent. The experience of having a caseworker perform what was essentially an interrogation of her postbirth is another violation. Laila was in need of someone supportive to help her work through her myriad feelings. Instead, she received state intervention with the aim of removing her child from her. Once Laila processed what had happened, she determined she wanted to keep the baby, yet she didn't feel that she would be able to take her child home because she was being repeatedly questioned about her capacity to mother her child. What Laila's case demonstrates is the wide range of experience that surrounds childbirth. Many expecting mothers come into the hospital in their most vulnerable state. But in the case of Black mothers and birthing people, the medical staff, instead of partnering with patients, often partner with the state, resulting in the criminalizing of Black birth that is affirmed in statistical data and research on disparate reporting of Black parents to child welfare services, as referenced above.

Laila's situation highlights the pervasive practice of policing Black birth. Unfortunately, an illustration of even more drastic policing would take place just after the end of our storytelling research when baby Mila Jackson was taken from her family on March 28, 2023, mere days after being delivered via home birth on March 21, 2023.

POLICING HOME BIRTHS

> I feel hunted. We feel hunted.
> —Rodney and Temecia Jackson

Although home births are legal in Texas, they are still stigmatized in the medical space. In *Birthing Liberation: How Reproductive Justice Can Set Us Free,* Sabia Wade (who refers to herself as "the Black

Doula") laments the "exile of Granny midwives and the increase of childbirth as a colonized, industrialized, and medicalized process."[15] This medicalization leaves Black women and birthing people especially vulnerable to obstetric violence and poor health outcomes for mother and baby. Coined by Dana-Aín Davis and expanded upon by researchers and thinkers like Karen A. Scott and Sabia Wade, the term *obstetric violence* essentially refers to "harm inflicted during or in relation to pregnancy, childbearing, and the post-partum period. Such violence can be both interpersonal and structural, arising from the actions of health-care providers and also from broader political and economic arrangements that disproportionately harm marginalized populations."[16] These realities were exactly what the Jackson family were hoping to avoid. They sought out a home birth as a way to claim their power to draw on the traditions of granny midwives and doulas so that Temecia Jackson (the birth mother) and Mila (the baby) could realize the tenets of reproductive justice, primarily bodily autonomy and nurturance of children in safe and healthy conditions as well as communities. Through the support of their midwife, Dr. Cheryl Edinbyrd, they achieved that goal. Mila was born healthy and at home. However, when the Jackson family engaged the medical space, the beautiful experience of Mila's birth soon turned into a nightmare.

In an April 6, 2023, press conference, Temecia and Rodney Jackson shared with the world the devastating news that their baby, Mila, had been taken by child protective services (CPS) in Dallas, Texas, and that the state would not return her to their custody. The trouble had begun when the couple had taken Mila to Dr. Bhatt's office for a newborn checkup on March 24, 2023. There a nurse practitioner gave the baby a clean bill of health. But later that day their doctor, Dr. Anand Bhatt (who had not seen the child himself) phoned them to tell them that the baby had jaundice, with an elevated level of bilirubin that was potentially dangerous and required treatment. According to Temecia, the doctor told them that the jaundice could be treated in the hospital or at home according to certain criteria. Rodney and Temecia opted for home treatment and were given instructions on how to carry it out. They ordered the equipment for the recommended light therapy and were preparing to provide recommended nutritional therapy as well. They felt confident because of the support of their midwife, Dr. Cheryl Edinbyrd, who was continuing to provide care for the family during postpartum. But later Bhatt changed his instructions, despite the midwife's report of Mila's improvement, and advised that the couple take the child to a local hospital. They reaffirmed to him that they preferred home treatment, but that was not enough for Dr. Bhatt, who then reported them to CPS. Soon after the report, CPS came to the family home at 4:00 a.m., but the Jacksons twice denied them entry. Eventually they returned with a warrant, removing the baby from the home and arresting Rodney for attempting to prevent the execution of a civil process.

In the press conference, Temecia and Rodney described the many indignities they had endured. First, they shared the trauma of the taking of their baby, which they described as a kidnapping. Through tears, Temecia described the harrowing experience of being separated from her child and husband.[17] Rodney and Temecia had two older sons, and this experience upended and traumatized the whole family. The couple also shared that the name of the mother on the CPS paperwork was not Temecia but the name of someone who had prior history with CPS, a fact that likely exacerbated the situation. Temecia was literally unmothered in the CPS paperwork. To add insult to injury, CPS updated the documents in response but listed Rodney as the "alleged" father. The state had essentially endeavored to unmother Temecia and undermine her and Rodney's legitimacy as parents, but the press conference worked to offer a visual counterimage to the public and a counternarrative to the dehumanizing narrative that CPS and the court system had perpetuated. The couple's pain was palpable through the screen.

The targeting of these Black parents for having a home birth is just one contemporary instance of practices that have a long history. From slavery times onward, the state has broken up Black families by a variety of means. Systems like welfare and child protective services surveil and criminalize Black parents under the guise of support services. Dorothy Roberts explains that we should refer to these kinds of entities as family policing systems because they operate "by policing families, primarily by threatening to take their children away or tak[ing] them away. And it is a form of really massive state surveillance and investigation, disruption of families, even destruction of families."[18] For the Jackson family this was inherently how the system functioned. The investigation and surveillance of families, especially Black ones, who are disproportionately targeted by CPS, are perpetual and constant. The fact that the office handling baby Mila's case placed the wrong person's name as the mother on the paperwork is more than a clerical error: it speaks to the larger carelessness of a system purporting to care about the safety of children. On April 7, 2023, Dorothy Roberts commented on X about the unfolding case of the Jackson family: "Taking this couple's baby for having a home birth shows the ugly truth about family policing—it targets Black families; tears families apart; collaborates with cops; turns doctors into cops; endangers children; violates human rights. #TornApart #abolishCPS."

Roberts connects the workings of the family policing system to the taking of baby Mila and, importantly, shows how these systems turn doctors into cops working with these systems to police and separate families. This is precisely what Dr. Anand Bhatt did. He served as a collaborator with the family policing system instead of his patients, the Jackson family, further breaking down the trust of Black people in medical spaces.

Ironically, baby Mila was placed in a foster home but received limited care that was not on par with what her birth family had been giving her. The Jacksons shared that they were allowed only two brief visits with their daughter and that during both visits they were video-recorded. They described feeling baited and "hunted" by the state. The video recordings were an attempt, they felt, to gather further evidence to substantiate their alleged unfitness as parents. During their visits, they discovered that baby Mila was experiencing "fluid buildup" (akin to vaginal discharge) on her private areas and what appeared to be a vaginal irritation. They inquired about this and did not receive satisfactory responses. Temecia had also been expressing breast milk for baby Mila, but she could not receive confirmation that the baby had received it. The foster caregivers had been giving the baby formula, which went against Temecia and Rodney's desired nutritional standards for their child. The cumulative effect of these violations undoubtedly took a toll on the family and baby. The early years of a child's life are most critical, and being separated from a loving mother during this time has to have had an indelible impact on Mila. While it will take time to know the full impact of this experience on the family, the weathering that they have endured is evident and ongoing.

At the end of the press conference, the executive director of the Afiya Center, Marsha Jones, and the midwife, Dr. Cheryl Edinbyrd, spoke. Marsha Jones asserted powerfully, "The attack on Black families has to stop." Both Jones and Edinbyrd declared that what Mila needed was her mother. In an emotional plea to the audience, Edinbyrd explained that this issue affected everyone: "Today it's them, but anybody can be abused by the CPS system." Together, Jones and Edinbyrd offered a critical sociopolitical context for what had happened to the Jackson family. Just before the April 20, 2023, hearing where a court was to decide if baby Mila would be returned to the family, the court ruled that she could return home.[19] The victory was bittersweet. The family was excited to be reunited with their daughter, but the pain of their separation will take an incredible amount of time and effort to heal.

REMOTHERING

The Jackson family's experience is a surreal (but very real) illustration of the damage caused by the family policing system and highlights the importance of addressing the failures of this system in supporting families. The 2023 film *A Thousand and One* homes in on this issue, offering a creative meditation on the devastating impact of interlocking systems of oppression (namely policing, child welfare, and gentrification) on Black children and families. Directed by A.V. Rockwell and starring Teyana Taylor, the film centers on Inez (played by Taylor), a fiercely determined and unapologetic young mother who kidnaps her son, Terry, from the foster care system in New York City. Set over several years, from the early 1990s to the early 2000s, the story follows Inez and Terry as they build their lives in Harlem. Inez works to provide a stable home for Terry so that he can have a better future, but the overwhelming forces of the systemic policing of Black families prove difficult to overcome.

Inez's act of taking Terry's and her own destiny into her hands can be seen as a form of remothering that directly resists the long-standing practice of unmothering Black women. Remothering has been mostly theorized in the psychology and therapy space as an act of mothering oneself or being the kind of mother one didn't have. It is a form of healing childhood wounds. But Inez's experience as a Black woman gives this term and her act a different dimension. We learn in the film that Inez herself was a victim of family separation and grew up in foster care. When Terry asks her where her family is, she says, "My family's gone, boo."[20] In many ways she is remothering herself because she was separated from her mother as a child. However, her taking of Terry is also an attempt to wrest control from the state, which has denied Terry his mother. Both Inez and Terry are orphans torn apart from their families by the same system. Inez's work to mother Terry is reparative for both of them. *A Thousand and One* asks the critical question: What becomes possible when Black families are kept together and aren't punished for the effects of systemic inequality?

The film opens in prison with an implicit critique of the carceral state. It sets the tone for what follows, in that a thread of carcerality runs through the film. Inez is an inmate in Rikers Island Prison for "boosting," or retail crime such as shoplifting. This is another sign of her condition and the likely poverty that informs her actions. We see Inez styling someone's hair in her cell. She is complimenting her client, and they are engaged in friendly banter. In the background and off screen, we hear another inmate tell someone that she is pregnant. They are joyful. The inmate tells the pregnant inmate, "You gonna get bigger, your feet gone swell."[21] They both laugh, and we hear a guard disrupting them and threatening them with isolation. To hear their joy met with a threat from the police signals yet another form of isolating Black people from loving relationships. The system is designed to take their joy, so the officer must disrupt it. Moreover, by including the experience of an inmate becoming pregnant, the film brings to light the reality that prisons often hold pregnant women and birthing people. The intertwining of the discourses of carceral medicine and isolation comes into greater awareness through this narrative layer.

Once Inez is released, the film turns to an exploration of the difficulties of reentry into society after incarceration and the problems within the foster care system. Because Inez is a hairstylist, she is able to provide for herself in limited ways. Of course, she needs space to offer her services to clients and she needs a home. As she works through that process, she encounters Terry, the child from whom she has been separated. She looks on as he is cared for in public by his foster mother. The foster mother speaks to him and the other children in her care in cold and unloving tones, much to Inez's concern. Terry eventually sustains injuries in the custody of his foster mother and has to be hospitalized. Inez is his only visitor. During this time, Terry tells Inez about his earliest memory, of being abandoned on a street corner (he mistakenly believes by Inez, though at the time she does not contradict this). One night, in exasperation over his lack of care, she takes him from the hospital. After a few days, Terry asks her why no one is looking for him and she doesn't have a concrete answer. What these scenes demonstrate is Terry's orphanhood and lack of any viable extended community of people who are invested in his life. The foster care system is also critiqued. While Terry might be in what the state considers a better environment, he does not receive loving care.

Another dimension of critique that the film explores is the overarching criminalization of Black life in metropolitan areas like New York City. Between the action scenes in the film are interludes of reporters sharing news developments in the city. We hear the voice of former New York City mayor Rudy Giuliani, who lauds the city's stop-and-frisk program responsible for the harassment and terror of Black citizens. A headline about the brutal attack of Abner Louima by New York City police crosses the screen.[22] While these events are announced, we also see Inez and Terry moving from place to place surreptitiously, in hiding from the carceral gaze. The viewer gets the sense that they are trying to avoid being hunted, the condition described by the Jacksons in their narrative about the state's effort to prove them to be unfit parents.

In spite of the practices informed by systemic racism swirling around Inez and Terry, they are able to build a life and have a semblance of stability. This work to build a life becomes the project of Inez's boyfriend Lucky, who was recently released from prison and is reconnecting with his loved ones. Lucky proves to be an unlikely anchor for Terry. Although he is hesitant to be a part of Inez's act of taking Terry from the hospital and living practically underground, he loves Inez and works with her to make a home. He jokes with Inez, "What do two crooks know about raising a family?"[23] That is indeed what they do, however. He marries Inez and declares to Terry, "We blood now. Nobody's going anywhere from this point on. I promise to protect you and your mother. We're gonna give you the life we never had."[24] Lucky's words are a promise and an Afrofuturist speculative form of resistance. His name, Lucky, holds irony because in so many respects he has been unlucky in his life, but in Terry he sees new possibility and a chance to rewrite the future that the state has for children like Terry.

To achieve the feat of giving Terry a life they have never had, Inez has to secure fake records for Terry to enroll in school. She gives him the name Darryl Terry Raymond and instructs him to tell people to go by his middle name as a way to align his past identity with his future one. Terry proves to be successful in school. He is a high-performing student, so much so that he is approached to apply to one of the top high schools in the city. He gets into that high school, and life appears to be looking up for the family. However, as Terry's life improves, the family's homelife gets worse. Lucky is diagnosed with cancer. Though his official age is unclear, his diagnosis comes at a relatively young age—likely his thirties or early forties. Inez and Terry regularly visit him in the hospital as he talks to them in raspy tones, his health slowly deteriorating. Again, weathering comes into play. For young men like Lucky, socioeconomic conditions and the afterlives of slavery lead to premature death. The film brings to light the fragility of Black life during these times. On his deathbed, Lucky counsels Terry about choosing a college. He tells him, "Go somewhere far. In my era, we didn't get those kind of shots."[25] Even as he is facing death, Lucky dreams of a brighter future for Terry. He knows that the present conditions in New York won't produce positive outcomes for Terry because they did not for him. In additional scenes between his visits to the hospital, we see Terry being stopped and frisked by police. Increasingly, he is encountering the carceral system, and this is intensifying as he grows older. Lucky wants Terry to change his environment and realize a potential elsewhere.

Lucky's death is the first thread of the family's self-woven fabric to unravel, signaling almost an impossibility of escaping the overwhelming forces of systemic oppression for Black people.

After Lucky dies, the apartment that Inez rents begins to have problems. It had recently been purchased by a new owner aiming to gentrify the area. Once the new owner takes over the property, things begin to malfunction (the stove, the water, basic necessities to make the home habitable). The owner tells Inez that making the repairs will require Inez to move out, but Inez senses that if she moves out she will be unable to move back in. So she stays through the harsh conditions, determined not to let the life she has built crumble. At the same time, however, Terry is applying to colleges and needs to produce a birth certificate and Social Security card. It is then that he learns from social services that his identity is a fake one and that Inez is actually not his mother at all. This is devastating to him. Having not known his birth mother, he has believed and trusted that Inez was his mother. Disillusioned, desperate for answers, and feeling alone, he asks her, "Where is home for me now?"[26]

Inez is defiant about her choice to take Terry and to raise him. Her reasoning shows her savvy in detecting the flaws of the family policing system and giving Terry a chance at life that he likely wouldn't have had in foster care. Research shows that children experience poor life outcomes once they are placed in the custody of the family policing system. Dorothy Roberts explains, "The claim that foster care improves Black children's welfare has been demolished by recent research. The evidence is clear that putting children in the foster care system is itself harmful. . . . Foster care magnifies the societal barriers and assaults that Black children already face because of structural racism."[27] Children raised in foster care often experience problems in adaptive functioning and are more likely to be entangled in the carceral web of juvenile detention and eventually imprisonment, according to Roberts.[28] Inez knows this firsthand because she was a victim of it herself.

In defense of herself and her efforts to save Terry from this fate, she explains to him, "I never left you on that corner. I was the one who found you. . . . I just wanted to look out for you. I seen somebody who needed me, but maybe I'm the one who needed you."[29] In this revealing moment, Inez not only shares her role in taking Terry to care for him, but also tells him that this act was probably a form of saving her own life. Dealing with the isolation of having been a foster child with no real familial connections clearly has had a significant impact on her. Even though she is caught up in the carceral system, she leaves with a determination to make a better life for herself. However, the commentary of the film is that the social supports in place cannot facilitate that for her because they actually perpetuate the inequities that they are designed to address. Inez knows this and declares to Terry, "I won because I know you gone grow up to be somebody."[30] She is in a battle for her life against the oppressive forces converging on her. And in many ways she does win. Terry is an adult now and likely won't be held responsible for his false records, as he is still considered a kidnapping victim. The film ends with Inez, now on the run from the law for the "kidnapping," getting a taxi ride to an unknown destination, leaving Terry to figure out next steps. We do not know Terry's outcome, but we know that he has built relationships through school and peers that will likely support this next phase of his life's journey. In spite of all the uncertainty, the film offers an ambiguous ending that doesn't imply despair. After the dust settles, Terry's and Inez's will to survive is likely to support them as they navigate their lives.

A Thousand and One functions as a tale of the family policing system, its harms and the critical need to resist. The film sheds light on stories like Shani's, Laila's, and the Jackson family's. A pervasive criminalization of Black birth begins at the womb and continues after the child is born. It is critical for the medical system and child welfare services to address the anti-Blackness that leads to family separation. The collective sharing of these assaults on family structures is its own form of waterbreaking—opening up space for critique of these systems by those who have been violated. The narrative perpetuated about child welfare services is one that aligns with a savior discourse. The question that must be asked is, How many families are destroyed in the wake of the surveillance and criminalization of poverty as well as Blackness?

EPILOGUE

You Won't Break My Soul

Affirmation
Our souls will not be broken.

In June of 2022, our storytelling work had come to an end, temporally, but the echoings of what had been shared, the relationships made, and the healing being done were reverberating for all of us. We sent each other emails about how we could harness the power that had emerged from our work into more. We knew that Livable Black Futures needed to continue. I would listen to our playlists and process. Then, on June 20, 2022, artist Beyoncé released a new song, ending her nearly three-year pause since her last project, *Black Is King*. "Break My Soul" emerged during a time of high cultural tension. The Covid-19 pandemic had increased the use of remote work, and many were experiencing awakenings about our value systems, reevaluating our toxic cultures of overwork, and more (shout-out to Tricia Hersey and her incredible work with the Nap Ministry).[1] Tricia Hersey had not yet released her manifesto *Rest Is Resistance*,[2] which was published in October 2022, but her teachings and interviews had inspired many who were embracing the healing power of rest. Although we were two years out from the 2020 racial reckonings and the presidential election, those events were also heavy in the consciousness of the US body politic. Perhaps most critically, we were awaiting the *Dobbs v. Jackson* decision, which challenged the constitutionality of *Roe v. Wade*. We had been on guard since the May 2022 leaked draft opinion that essentially forecasted that Thomas E. Dobbs, state health officer of Mississippi's Department of Health, would prevail in the challenge to the state's law banning abortion after fifteen weeks of pregnancy that had been brought by Jackson Women's Health Organization and the Center for Reproductive Rights. The end of *Roe v. Wade* was in the air. Those of us living in states like Mississippi and Texas knew that if the Supreme Court ruled in favor of Dobbs, abortion would be illegal. They were trying to break our souls.

Beyoncé's "Break My Soul" was a call to birth something new out of struggle. The lyrics spoke to the work of Livable Black Futures on many levels. The song opens explosively like a waterbreaking, a force pushing forward to release and welcome in something new. Beyoncé enters the song with a different kind of intensity. It is melodic but determined. I think back to Daphne Brooks's assertion that Black women's musical practices "forecast and execute the viability and potentiality of Black life."[3] Beyoncé's declaration that no one will break her soul is a clear articulation of that viability in spite of all odds. Expansive in its reach and content, the song speaks to multiply marginalized people as a kind of anthem for self-determination in the face of oppression. The song immediately became a take-off hit at LGBTQ+ Pride events, abortion rallies, and anywhere people were organizing against oppression.[4] Seeing the way the song expressed our collective sentiments made me wish it had been released during our storytelling research, but in so many ways it was a nice coda to our work. It felt right that the song would be released after we were done. I can imagine each member of our storytelling group processing what it meant to them. To me, it was a call to keep going and to invest myself in soul-affirming rather than soul-crushing work—and to not be fearful of what was to come but to know that whatever came, it wouldn't break me or any of us fighting the fight for bodily autonomy and reproductive freedom.

"Break My Soul" demonstrates the power of Black feminist storytelling and how, no matter the form, using narrative to speak back to power holds great possibilities for personal and collective freedom. Throughout this work, I come back to the ways that sharing our unique and diverse stories enabled them to serve as vehicles of inspiration and healing. It was our own archive of medical experience separate from the medical record, which doesn't have the capacity to hold the humanity of our stories. I couldn't help but feel the symbolic resonance of the end of our storytelling journey for advancing reproductive freedom being synchronous with the fall of *Roe v. Wade*. However, rather than yield to despair, this reality increased my resolve to continue this work. Although most of this book has been about the fight to advance greater bodily autonomy and birthing liberation, the right to a safe abortion remains one of the biggest battles in our present era. We are seeing the damage of abortion bans and restrictive laws in states like Texas and Georgia, and they are affecting Black women and birthing people significantly. These laws, because of the ways they engender fear in women and birthing people, are creating greater isolation and more limitations on medical care, which can have deadly consequences.

BANS OFF OUR BODIES

Even though our storytelling research ended before the *Dobbs v. Jackson* decision, we had been dealing with the harbinger of the decision in the form of Texas's Senate Bill 8, the Heartbeat Bill, which banned abortion after six weeks or once a fetal heartbeat was detected. Our discussions yielded great insight into what people were contending with as they grappled with efforts to take away their reproductive freedom. One of our doulas and co-researchers was especially close to these realities because of her participation in the Afiya Center's abortion care work. She asserted, "They're trying to put bans on our bodies." Her words carry forward the discourse of the Bans Off Our Bodies campaign led by Planned Parenthood in coalition with other organizations working to advance reproductive freedom. The site explains the focus of the campaign: "Bans Off Our Bodies is a national abortion rights campaign. It is led by abortion rights supporters in response to unrelenting political attacks on our basic right to control our own bodies, our lives, and our futures."[5] This work has become increasingly crucial as the encroachment on the bodily autonomy of women and birthing people is ever increasing, from abortion bans to restrictions on gender-affirming care and more.

As our doulas raised discussion on this, more of our storytellers opened up. One person, Jade, talked about how even traveling out of state for an abortion was becoming more costly. She recalls the experience of a friend who needed an abortion but faced enormous barriers in doing so. Her friend wanted to travel to New Mexico for her abortion because she thought its closeness to Texas would make the cost relatively inexpensive, but her ticket was much more expensive than anticipated, totaling up to $400. The woman seeking the abortion also had to take her child with her because she didn't have childcare. She spent her limited funds getting her and her child to New Mexico for the abortion.

Many of our storytellers shared similar knowledges, expressing that people in their communities were concerned about the limited paths to receiving an abortion should they need one. They referred to it as forced birth—feeling trapped without options for themselves. Akina, another storyteller, shared an experience of having to visit a crisis pregnancy center (CPC) because so many Planned Parenthoods had closed in Texas. Interestingly, as Planned Parenthoods were facing closures in Texas, CPCs were on the rise. Planned Parenthood sounded the alarm about CPCs in a statement issued in 2021. They warned, "Crisis pregnancy centers (also called CPCs or 'fake clinics') are clinics or mobile vans that look like real health centers, but they're run by anti-abortion activists who have a shady, harmful agenda: to scare, shame, or pressure you out of getting an abortion, and to tell lies about abortion, birth control, and sexual health."[6] This description aligns with the experiences our storytellers reported among those who, in desperation, sought out a crisis pregnancy center for an abortion.

At the CPC she visited, Akina met with numerous challenges to receiving abortion care. She thought she was four weeks pregnant, but they said her ultrasound said seven weeks, just outside of the window of time in which she could receive an abortion. And even if she had been counted at four weeks, they shared that it would take about two weeks to schedule an appointment with a doctor who could facilitate her abortion, again placing her outside of the legal window. More than that, they tried to persuade her to keep her baby or consider adoption, and they provided other forms of moralizing that she had not anticipated. She declared, "Don't project your morals onto me. I'm here for a service." She also shared her concern about women in abusive relationships who were seeking abortion as a way out and how these CPCs were limiting their ability to escape abusive situations.

In addition to the barriers to abortion facing us in Texas, our storytellers expressed concern about what these developments would mean for the criminalization of Black women and birthing people who were already navigating the criminalizing gaze of anti-Blackness and misogynoir. We were seeing this in real time with cases like that of Lizelle Herrera, a twenty-six-year-old woman in South Texas who was charged with murder when Texas officials alleged that she had caused the death of an individual by self-induced abortion. Herrera took the legal drug misoprostol to end her pregnancy and had subsequent treatment at a local hospital to remove the fetus. Medical staff at the hospital reported the abortion, which led to her arrest.[7] Herrera being a woman of color underscores the way these laws add another layer of criminality to those already viewed through this lens. Herrera was ultimately not tried for murder, but the trauma of the experience remains with her. She is currently suing the state for damages.

There are also concerns about what it means to be forced to carry nonviable or life-threatening fetuses because of the abortion ban. Kate Cox, thirty-one years old and also from Texas, sued unsuccessfully for the right to abort a nonviable pregnancy in 2023. The fetus had full trisomy 18, a lethal fetal anomaly. She sought an abortion for this situation, but doctors refused to perform it because of state prohibitions against abortion. This meant she had to travel to another state to have the procedure, which also put her life in danger.[8] This case raises serious causes for concern for patients and medical professionals alike. In the cases of Herrera and Cox, we see a breakdown of relationships between medical providers and the vulnerable patients in their care. Moreover, the abortion bans empower intrusive providers to violate the trust and rights of their patients to privacy and care. Unfortunately, these Texas cases have been just the beginning of the fallout of the harmful abortion bans brought on by the *Dobbs v. Jackson* decision. The stories of Amber Thurman and Candi Miller, also victims of state restrictions on abortion, demonstrate the deadly implications of these bans. Although both women have passed away, they remind us of why we fight and why we must tell our stories.

A PREVENTABLE CRISIS

In the aftermath of restrictive abortion bans across the US South, women are dying, particularly Black women. Afiya Center executive director Marsha Jones sounded the alarm about this potential in a June 2024 interview. "So much harm could happen," Jones said. "We can't step away from the dangers of birthing as a Black person, especially in the South. It is real. . . . The Dobbs decision has really magnified the gaps that are there and increased them with no solution."[9] Black women and birthing people have been contending with the Black perinatal health crisis for many years, and these new developments add to the dangers. Yet the deaths resulting from that crisis and the bans on abortion are preventable. The crisis is manmade.

The case of twenty-eight-year-old Georgia woman Amber Thurman highlights the deadly results of the gaps in care that are emerging out of the *Dobbs v. Jackson* decision. Amber Thurman died from lack of care following her use of mifepristone, medication abortion.[10] Thurman was an aspiring nurse and mother of a six-year-old son. She became pregnant in 2022 and was not ready to have a second child. She traveled to North Carolina in August 2022 for abortion support and received mifepristone from a provider. She took the mifepristone but needed a D&C (a dilation and curettage) procedure to expel the remaining fetal tissue. Because of Georgia's prohibitive laws, doctors could not remove the fetal tissue from Thurman's body until her life was in danger. However, by then it was too late. She went into septic shock and died in August 2022. Her last words to her mother were a plea to take care of her son.

According to ProPublica, a group of medical experts determined that Thurman did not have to die. "Tasked with examining pregnancy-related deaths to improve maternal health, the experts [examining the case], including 10 doctors, deemed hers 'preventable' and said the hospital's delay in performing the critical procedure had a 'large' impact on her fatal outcome."[11] Abortion bans have put medical providers in the difficult position of delaying care until it is too late. Medical experts confirm that the language of exceptions to protect the "life of the mother" is not sufficient to address the realities of medicine, including the subjective and slippery nature of that concept. More than that, doctors have become cautious to an extreme to avoid criminal punishment for supporting women and birthing people needing to end pregnancies for varying reasons.

> Doctors in public hospitals and those outside of major metro areas told ProPublica that they are often left scrambling to figure out on a case-by-case basis when they are allowed to provide D&Cs and other abortion procedures. Many fear they are taking on all of the risk

alone and would not be backed up by their hospitals if a prosecutor charged them with a crime. At Catholic hospitals, they typically have to transfer patients elsewhere for care.[12]

Increasingly, oppressive laws and an already carceral underpinning of medicine (in the form of surveillance and criminalization, particularly in the case of Black patients) distance doctors from their patients and prevent the development of a collaborative care relationship. Doctors are positioned more on the side of the state than on the side of the patient.

The criminalization of abortion and the fear of seeking help are what led to the death of Candi Miller in November 2022.[13] A forty-one-year-old wife and mother of three, Candi Miller unintentionally got pregnant, and her health situation—diagnoses of lupus, diabetes, and hypertension—created complications for proceeding with the pregnancy. Miller knew that she needed to act because her advanced maternal age and her comorbidities could prove deadly for her. Because of Georgia's oppressive laws, she feared being criminalized for having an abortion, so she sought one on her own, which is something abortion rights advocates have warned would be the outcome of abortion bans. Miller needed medical supervision but was afraid to seek it. Her family later told a coroner she hadn't visited a doctor "due to the current legislation on pregnancies and abortions."[14] She had been experiencing not only increasing health concerns relating to her pregnancy but also mental health concerns. She isolated herself, and anxiety and depression had a deep impact on her. I think about the life-giving work of our storytelling circles and how so many of our storytellers spoke of the positive effects of being able to have shame-free conversations about their sexual and reproductive health in supportive spaces. It is also important to note that exceptions made for abortion do not include the mental health of the mother.

> The exceptions are limited to acute emergencies, usually defined as when "necessary in order to prevent the death of the pregnant woman or the substantial and irreversible physical impairment of a major bodily function." They also specifically prohibit mental health reasons from counting as health emergencies, even if a pregnant woman says she is thinking about harming herself. In Georgia, violating the law can cost doctors their license and subject them to prison terms of up to 10 years.[15]

What the state of Georgia has done with these kinds of restrictions is issue a death sentence for many women and birthing people who for varying reasons cannot sustain a pregnancy. They should have the option to determine what is the best path for them instead of the state forcing them to carry a pregnancy to term.

Amber Thurman's and Candi Miller's deaths have ignited a national conversation about the deadly impact of the *Dobbs v. Jackson* decision and the abortion bans across the South. The Feminist Women's Health Center in Georgia offers a powerful encapsulation of the injustice of Thurman's and Miller's deaths. They state:

> These women did not die because of the medications they took. They died because of the gross negligence of the providers they sought for help. They died because of the confusing and ambiguous language included in the law. They died because of fear of criminalization—both their own in the case of Candi Miller, who suffered at home because she was afraid to seek care under the confusing abortion law, and that of the healthcare providers who refused to act on Amber's behalf.[16]

Amber Thurman and Candi Miller's deaths were preventable. It is critical to say their names as often as we can to amplify what is at stake in the fight for abortion and bodily autonomy. No one should be forced to carry a pregnancy, and no one should die because they cannot or do not want to carry a pregnancy to term.

"ME REPLACED BY WE": A WORD FROM ASSATA

I end this book with Assata Shakur's words, since her articulation of the importance of resisting for a better world underscores my hopes for this book and how it might engender more storytelling as a practice of freedom. When we break the silence of our experiences, we are giving others a road map for resistance. Telling our stories in whatever form they might take is most critical today as structural forces aim to isolate women and birthing people from each other and arguably their own bodies. Assata Shakur's poem "Love," in which she declares: "We are pregnant with freedom/ We are a conspiracy," is both a declaration and a prayer. It signals a possible world that we might create out of oppression. The imagining of possible futures is deeply needed. By engaging with the work of the Black gynecological publics (Black writers, activists, advocates, artists, and community members), I located stories that speak powerfully to ongoing issues of medical injustice, abortion, and the need to enact care that supports everyone, regardless of their identity or proximity to resources. Their work affirms that Black feminist storytelling serves as a key site for advancing and expanding the underlying tenets of reproductive justice.

The ending of *Assata* represents the collective work I witnessed to prioritize the "We" in our society and to dream amid despair. *Assata* comes full circle when, at the end of the work, Shakur is grappling with how to achieve freedom and mother her daughter Kakuya. Although Kakuya was conceived with intention and birthed in love, the separation from her mother took a toll on their relationship. She would visit and be hostile to her mother—angry about her imprisonment. She told her mother, "You can get out of here if you want to. . . . You just don't want to."[17] Kakuya told her grandmother to instruct Assata to open the bars. Assata invited Kakuya to try, and she tried to no avail. After this visit, Assata cried until she vomited but resolved to get free. It was her daughter's rage that reignited her will to resist. She wanted to feel what it was like to mother outside of the bars. Near the end of her autobiography, she offers a poem to Kakuya:

To My Daughter Kakuya
Assata Shakur

i have shabby dreams for you
of some vague freedom
i have never known.

Baby,
i don't want you hungry or thirsty
or out in the cold.
and i don't want the frost
to kill your fruit
before it ripens.

i can see a sunny place—
Life exploding green.
i can see your bright, bronze skin at ease with all the flowers
and the centipedes.

i can hear laughter,
not grown from ridicule
And words not prompted
by ego or greed or jealousy.

i see a world where hatred
has been replaced by love.
and ME replaced by WE.

And I can see a world replaced
where you,
building and exploring,
strong and fulfilled,
will understand.

And go beyond
my little shabby dreams.[18]

In this poem, Assata is still learning how to dream again. The carceral system has steadily worked on her, aiming to break her spirit and her resolve to resist racism and holistic oppression. It is through Kakuya that she sees possibility and hope for a better world—a ME replaced by WE. In a 1988 interview with Cheryll Greene, Shakur talks about what it has been like to reunite with Kakuya in Cuba and raise her. She shares how inspired she is by her daughter and how quick she was to learn Spanish. She looks to her daughter and her generation to enact bigger freedom dreams. "She has had a chance to really see and be exposed to the struggles of other people here, to see that life can be better and that people can take action to change their life."[19] Kakuya is pregnant with freedom. She is able to see the possibilities for a better world and has the opportunity to live out the "shabby dreams" (which are not at all shabby) that her mother has for her.

I think about what it means to create the kind of world that Assata dreams of for Kakuya and make that possible for all people. The storytelling work I've engaged in is one form of me exploring this query. I also draw on the legacies of Black feminist revolutionaries who did not accept the world as it was but dreamed of (and worked to make possible) the world as it could be. It is this sentiment that Monica Simpson, executive director of SisterSong, expresses when she says: "They [Harriet Tubman and freedom fighters of the civil rights movement] literally had to think outside of what was in front of them. . . . [We have to be] willing to make ourselves uncomfortable in order to see something better than what's in front of us."[20] The collective resistance emerging in different parts of the country signals this. In our part of the world, we are using storytelling as a way to tap into that consciousness and birth new realities. As I think of where we go from here, it is unclear what is next, but Marsha Jones expresses what those of us involved in this work feel: "We really won't stop."[21] We are pregnant with freedom indeed.

CODA

I completed the writing of this book before the 2024 presidential election in the United States. Although I anticipated further retrenchment of reproductive freedom and racial justice, I have been deeply troubled by the fact that language has been the primary site of contestation even as I have spent much of this book exploring the power of language. Words such as *diversity, equity,* and *inclusion* are deemed illegal. Those applying for grants from the National Institutes of Health and the National Science Foundation have been urged to avoid liberatory language such as *accessibility, advocacy, bias, race,* and any words signaling health inequity.

More than anything, these assaults on language demonstrate the power of our stories to enact change. A major challenge for the work of reproductive justice and justice more broadly is to resist the silencing of our voices. We must also create spaces that are not wholly dependent on government funding so that the work continues, as it desperately needs to. This means that we lean into community more. That we tap into our imaginations as tools of resistance. While we work for structural change, we must correspondingly reclaim our power to birth new worlds through our stories that cannot be undone or erased.

NOTES

FOREWORD

1. The Livable Black Futures Collective uses terms such as *womxn* and *wombholders* as a way to name all those affected by gynecological and obstetric medicine (inclusive of womxn, trans, and nonbinary folks).

2. Senate Bill 8, Texas State Senate, May 13, 2021, https://capitol.texas.gov/tlodocs/87R/billtext/pdf/SB00008F.pdf.

3. Donna L. Hoyert, "Maternal Mortality Rates in the United States, 2020," Centers for Disease Control and Prevention, February 23, 2022, www.cdc.gov/nchs/data/hestat/maternal-mortality/2020/maternal-mortality-rates-2020.htm.

4. Audre Lorde, "Man Child: A Black Lesbian Feminist's Response," in *Zami; Sister Outsider; Undersong* (Mechanicsburg, PA: Quality Paperback Book Club, 1993), 74.

5. Dorothy Roberts, *Killing the Black Body: Race, Reproduction, and the Meaning of Liberty* (New York: Pantheon Books, 1997), 23.

6. Combahee River Collective, *The Combahee River Collective Statement* (1977), reprinted as a reading on Yale University's American Studies website, https://americanstudies.yale.edu/sites/default/files/files/Keyword%20Coalition_Readings.pdf.

7. Afiya Center, 15th Anniversary booklet, 2023, in author's private collection.

8. Afiya Center, 15th Anniversary booklet, 2023.

9. Whole Woman's Health v. Austin R. Jackson, Case 1:21-cv-00616 (US District Court—Austin Division 2021), Complaint for Declaratory and Injunctive Relief — Class Action, July 2021, https://reproductiverights.org/wp-content/uploads/2021/07/WWH-v.-Jackson-Complaint.pdf.

10. See Venus E. Evans-Winters, *Black Feminism in Qualitative Inquiry: A Mosaic for Writing Our Daughter's Body* (London: Routledge, 2019), and S.R. Toliver, *Recovering Black Storytelling in Qualitative Research: Endarkened Storywork* (New York: Routledge, 2022).

11. Byllye Avery, "Empowerment through Wellness," *Yale Journal of Law and Feminism* 4 (1991): 147, https://heinonline.org/HOL/LandingPage?handle=hein.journals/yjfem4&div=18&id=&page=.

12. Robin D.G. Kelley, *Freedom Dreams: The Black Radical Imagination* (Boston: Beacon Press, 2003), 8.

INTRODUCTION

1. Dobbs v. Jackson Women's Health Organization, *SCOTUS Blog*, 2021, www.scotusblog.com/case-files/cases/dobbs-v-jackson-womens-health-organization/.

2. Glenn C. Altschuler, "Six Reasons Why Moms for Liberty Is an Extremist Organization," *The Hill*, July 9, 2023, https://thehill.com/opinion/education/4086179-six-reasons-why-moms-for-liberty-is-an-extremist-organization/.

3. Students for Fair Admissions, Inc. v. President and Fellows of Harvard College, Docket 20–1199 (1st Circuit Court 2023), www.scotusblog.com/case-files/cases/students-for-fair-admissions-inc-v-president-fellows-of-harvard-college/.

4. Marcela Rodriguez, "Gov. Abbott Signs DEI Bill into Law, Dismantling Diversity Offices at Colleges," *Dallas Morning News*, June 14, 2023, www.dallasnews.com/news/education/2023/06/14

/gov-abbott-signs-dei-bill-into-law-dismantling-diversity-offices-at-colleges/.

5. "Reproductive Justice," SisterSong, accessed March 10, 2023, www.sistersong.net/reproductive-justice.

6. See Loretta J. Ross, "Conceptualizing Reproductive Justice Theory: A Manifesto for Activism," in *Radical Reproductive Justice: Foundation, Theory, Practice, Critique*, ed. Loretta J. Ross et al. (New York: Feminist Press, 2017), 203.

7. See Lorretta J. Ross and Rickie Solinger, *Reproductive Justice: An Introduction* (Oakland: University of California Press, 2017), 59.

8. See Robin D.G. Kelley's *Freedom Dreams: The Black Radical Imagination* (Boston: Beacon Press, 2003).

9. See Monika Thakur, Suzanne M. Jenkins, and Kunal Mahajan, "Cervical Insufficiency," StatPearls, National Library of Medicine, October 6, 2024, www.ncbi.nlm.nih.gov/books/NBK525954/.

10. "Fannie Lou Hamer," PBS, accessed March 10, 2024, www.pbs.org/wgbh/americanexperience/features/freedomsummer-hamer/.

11. See Audre Lorde, "Man Child: A Black Lesbian Feminist's Response," in *Zami; Sister Outsider; Undersong* (Mechanicsburg, PA: Quality Paperback Book Club, 1993), 74.

12. Quoted in Cara Page, Erica Woodland, and Aurora Levins Morales, *Healing Justice Lineages: Dreaming at the Crossroads of Liberation, Collective Care, and Safety* (Berkeley, CA: North Atlantic Books, 2023), 103.

13. See Ross and Solinger, *Reproductive Justice*.

14. See S.R. Toliver, *Recovering Black Storytelling in Qualitative Research: Endarkened Storywork* (New York: Routledge, 2022).

15. Quoted in Stephanie Y. Evans et al., "Introduction: Race, Gender, and Public Health: Social Justice and Wellness Work," in *Black Women and Public Health: Strategies to Name, Locate and Change Systems of Power*, ed. Stephanie Y. Evans et al. (Albany: State University of New York Press, 2022), 23.

16. Toliver, *Recovering Black Storytelling*, xviii.

17. Karen A. Scott, Laura Britton, and Monica R. McLemore, "The Ethics of Perinatal Care for Black Women: Dismantling the

Structural Racism in 'Mother Blame' Narratives," *Journal of Perinatal and Neonatal Nursing* 33, no. 2 (2019): 108–15.

18. Monica R. McLemore and Esther K. Choo, "The Right Decisions Need the Right Voices," *The Lancet* 394, no. 10204 (2019): 1113–1204.

19. Sue Sturgis, "Is a Duke Energy Power Plant Making Nearby Residents Sick?," *Facing South*, May 1, 2014, www.facingsouth.org/2014/05/is-a-duke-energy-power-plant-making-nearby-residen.html.

20. Julie Bosman, "After Water Fiasco, Trust in Officials Is in Short Supply in Flint," *New York Times*, October 8, 2016, www.nytimes.com/2016/10/09/us/after-water-fiasco-trust-of-officials-is-in-short-supply-in-flint.html.

21. "Mississippi City's Water Problems Stem from Generations of Neglect," Southern Poverty Law Center, June 28, 2023, www.splcenter.org/news/2023/06/28/timeline-jackson-mississippi-water-problems#:~:text=Mississippi%20city's%20water%20problems%20stem%20from%20generations%20of%20neglect&text=On%20Aug.,no%20water%20service%20at%20all.

22. "Katrina Victims Blame Racism for Slow Aid," *NBC News*, December 6, 2005, www.nbcnews.com/id/wbna10354221.

23. Amanishakete Ani, "C-Section and Racism: 'Cutting' to the Heart of the Issue for Black Women and Families," *Journal of African American Studies* 19, no. 4 (2015): 343–61, https://doi.org/10.1007/s12111-015-9310-4.

24. Assata Shakur, *Assata: An Autobiography* (Chicago: Lawrence Hill Books, 2001), 93.

25. Shakur, *Assata*, 130.

26. Saidiya Hartman, *Lose Your Mother: A Journey along the Atlantic Slave Route* (New York: Farrar, Straus, and Giroux, 2007), 6.

27. Shakur, *Assata*, 180.

28. Venus E. Evans-Winters, *Black Feminism in Qualitative Inquiry: A Mosaic for Writing Our Daughter's Body* (London: Routledge, 2019), 16.

29. Toni Morrison, "The Site of Memory," in *Inventing the Truth: The Art and Craft of Memoir*, ed. William Zinsser (New York: Houghton Mifflin, 1995), 85–102.

30. Gayatri Spivak, "Can the Subaltern Speak?," in *Marxism and the Interpretation of Culture*, ed. Cary Nelson and Lawrence Grossberg (Champaign-Urbana: University of Illinois Press, 1988), 271–313.

31. Hartman, *Lose Your Mother*, 12.

32. See Deirdre Cooper Owens's *Medical Bondage: Race, Gender, and the Origins of American Gynecology* (Albany: University of Georgia Press, 2017) and Harriet Washington's *Medical Apartheid: The Dark History of Medical Experimentation on Black Americans from Colonial Times to the Present* (New York: Knopf Doubleday, 2008).

33. Hartman, *Lose Your Mother*, 13.

34. Combahee River Collective, *The Combahee River Collective Statement* (1977), reprinted as a reading on Yale University's American Studies website, https://americanstudies.yale.edu/sites/default/files/files/Keyword%20Coalition_Readings.pdf.

35. Ross, "Conceptualizing Reproductive Justice Theory," 173.

36. To be sure, these groups are not meant to typify those who are in reproductive justice movements—though reproductive justice can often attract people invested in the gender binary.

37. See Treva B. Lindsey, *America, Goddam: Violence, Black Women, and the Struggle for Justice* (Oakland: University of California Press, 2023).

38. Toni Morrison, *Beloved* (New York: Alfred A. Knopf, 1987), 51.

1. TOWARD A RADICAL *WE*

1. Campbell adapts this term from Valerie Purdie-Vaughns and Richard P. Eibach, "Intersectional Invisibility: The Distinctive Advantages and Disadvantages of Multiple Subordinate-Group Identities," *Sex Roles* 59 (2008): 377–91, https://doi.org/10.1007/s11199-008-9424-4.

2. Kai M. Green, "The Essential I/Eye in We: A Black Transfeminist Approach to Ethnographic Film," *Black Camera: An International Film Journal*, n.s., 6, no. 2 (2015): 196, https://doi.org/10.2979/blackcamera.6.2.187.

3. Fannie Lou Hamer, "Nobody's Free until Everybody's Free. Speech Delivered at the Founding of the National Women's Political Caucus, Washington, DC, July 10, 1971," in *The Speeches of Fannie Lou Hamer: To Tell It Like It Is*, ed. Maegan Parker Brooks and Davis W. Houck (Jackson: University Press of Mississippi, 2010), 134–39.

4. Ericka Hart, "My Birthing Experience as a Black, Queer Parent Was Traumatic and—against All Odds—Joyful," *Refinery29*, April 13, 2013, www.refinery29.com/en-us/2023/04/11357620/ericka-hart-black-birthing-story-queer-parenting.

5. Nancy Lapid, "U.S. Maternal Mortality More Than Doubled since 1999, Most Deaths among Black Women, Study Says," Reuters, July 3, 2023, www.reuters.com/world/us/us-maternal-mortality-more-than-doubled-since-1999-most-deaths-among-black-women-2023-07-03/.

6. "What Is Birth Justice?" Voices for Birth Justice, accessed June 19, 2022, https://voicesforbirthjustice.org/birth-justice/.

7. Sagaree Jain, "Two-Eyed Seeing: Decolonizing Methodologies for Reproductive Justice," *AMPLIFY*, May 19, 2020, https://medium.com/amplify/two-eyed-seeing-decolonizing-methodologies-for-reproductive-justice-ca16578e9e4a.

8. S.R. Toliver, *Recovering Black Storytelling in Qualitative Research: Endarkened Storywork* (New York: Routledge, 2022), xxxii.

9. Eve Purdy, "Embracing Messiness in Medicine, Research, and Ourselves," *ICE Blog: International Clinician Educators*, January 22, 2019, https://icenet.blog/2019/01/22/embracing-messiness-in-medicine-research-and-ourselves/.

10. See Treva B. Lindsey, *America, Goddam: Violence, Black Women, and the Struggle for Justice* (Oakland: University of California Press, 2023), 18.

11. Lindsey, *America, Goddam*, 151.

12. WFAA Staff, "No Indictment in Case of Dallas Woman Who Died after Being Restrained by Police," *WFAA*, May 12, 2023,

www.wfaa.com/article/news/local/dee-dee-hall-death-dallas-texas-investigation-police-grand-jury-indictment/287-8c9a35c4-e2fe-4517-89cf-650d3329190d.

13. Maria Guerrero, "Family of Transgender Woman Who Died in Dallas Police Custody Speak Out," *NBC 5 Dallas-Fort Worth*, June 13, 2022, www.nbcdfw.com/news/local/family-of-transgender-woman-who-died-in-dallas-police-custody-speak-out/2991447/.

14. Esther Kaner, "Abolition Medicine: Dismantling Carceral Logics in Healthcare," National Survivor User Network, December 15, 2021, www.nsun.org.uk/abolition-medicine-dismantling-carceral-logics-in-healthcare/.

15. Audre Lorde, "The Master's Tools Will Never Dismantle the Master's House," in *Zami; Sister Outsider; Undersong* (Mechanicsburg, PA: Quality Paperback Book Club, 1993), 112.

16. Cullen Peele, "Roundup of Anti-LGBTQ+ Legislation Advancing in States across the Country," Human Rights Campaign, press release, May 23, 2023, www.hrc.org/press-releases/roundup-of-anti-lgbtq-legislation-advancing-in-states-across-the-country.

17. Matt Lavietes, "Over Half of 2022's Most Challenged Books Have LGBTQ Themes," *NBC News*, April 25, 2023, www.nbcnews.com/nbc-out/out-politics-and-policy/half-2022s-challenged-books-lgbtq-themes-rcna81324.

18. Joe Hernandez, "Target Removes Some Pride Month Products after Threats against Employees," *NPR*, May 24, 2023, www.npr.org/2023/05/24/1177963864/target-pride-month-lgbtq-products-threats.

19. Veronica Barcelona et al., "Adverse Pregnancy and Birth Outcomes in Sexual Minority Women from the National Survey of Family Growth," *BMC Pregnancy and Childbirth* 22, no. 1 (2022): 923, https://doi.org/10.1186/s12884-022-05271-0.

20. Shabab Ahmed Mirza and Caitlin Rooney, "Discrimination Prevents LGBTQ People from Accessing Health Care," Center for American Progress, August 23, 2022, www.americanprogress.org/article/discrimination-prevents-lgbtq-people-accessing-health-care/.

21. Shannon Firth, "Anti-gay Stigma Shortens Lives," *U.S. News and World Report*, February 19, 2014, www.usnews.com/news/articles/2014/02/19/research-anti-gay-stigma-shortens-lives.

22. KB Brookins, "Sexting at the Gynecologist," *Poets Reading the News*, May 19, 2021, www.poetsreadingthenews.com/2021/05/sexting-at-the-gynecologist/.

23. KB Brookins, "This Is What It's Like Going to the Gynecologist When You're Black, Trans and in Texas," *HuffPost*, February 10, 2022, www.huffpost.com/entry/black-trans-texas-abortion-gynecologist_n_61f7fe58e4b04f9a12c06a7a.

24. Rebecca Dekker, host, "Black-Led Queer and Trans Birth Work with Mystique Hargrove, Kortney Lapeyrolerie, and Nadine Ashby," Episode 182 of *Evidence Based Birth* podcast, July 28, 2023, https://evidencebasedbirth.com/black-led-queer-and-trans-birth-work-with-mystique-hargrove-kortney-lapeyrolerie-and-nadine-ashby/.

25. Faith Karimi and Natalie Johnson, "A Woman Left the ER to Find Another Hospital after a Long Wait. Two Hours Later, She Was Dead." *CNN*, January 17, 2020, www.cnn.com/2020/01/17/us/tashonna-ward-death-questions-trnd/index.html.

26. See Deirdre Cooper Owens, *Medical Bondage: Race, Gender, and the Origins of American Gynecology* (Albany: University of Georgia Press, 2017).

27. Heidi L. Janz, "Ableism: The Undiagnosed Malady Afflicting Medicine," *Canadian Medical Association Journal* 191, no. 17 (2019): E478–E479, https://doi.org/10.1503/cmaj.180903.

28. Therí Pickens, "'You're Supposed to Be a Tall, Handsome, Fully Grown White Man': Theorizing Race, Gender, and Disability in Octavia Butler's *Fledgling*," *Journal of Literary and Cultural Disability Studies* 8, no. 1 (2014): 34, https://doi.org/10.3828/jlcds.2014.3.

29. To learn more about Robin Wilson-Beattie, see her website: www.robinwb.com.

30. Robin Wilson-Beattie, "My Abortion Story," Disability Visibility Project blog, July 28, 2015, https://disabilityvisibilityproject.com/2015/07/28/guest-blog-post-by-robin-wilson-beattie-my-abortion-story/#:~:text=Robin%3A%20My%20story%20actually%20starts,really%20grueling%20pregnancy%20with%20her.

31. Tien Sydnor-Campbell, "Sex, Sexuality, and the Disabled Black Woman," *Journal of Black Sexuality and Relationships* 3, no. 3 (2017): 67, https://dx.doi.org/10.1353/bsr.2017.0004.

32. Linda Villarosa, "The Long Shadow of Eugenics in America," *New York Times Magazine*, June 8, 2022, www.nytimes.com/2022/06/08/magazine/eugenics-movement-america.html; Mary Crossley, "Reproducing Dignity: Race, Disability, and Reproductive Controls," *U.C. Davis Law Review* 54 (Spring 2020).

33. Loretta J. Ross, "Trust Black Women: Reproductive Justice and Eugenics," in *Radical Reproductive Justice: Foundation, Theory, Practice, Critique*, ed. Loretta J. Ross et al. (New York: Feminist Press, 2017), 59.

34. Ross, "Trust Black Women," 69.

35. Carlos Nesbeth et al., "HIV Mortality Difference between Black and White Women," *Journal of Health Disparities Research and Practice* 11, no. 1 (2018): 179–90, https://digitalscholarship.unlv.edu/cgi/viewcontent.cgi?article=1699&context=jhdrp#:~:text=In%20these%20descriptive%20data%20from,that%20of%20their%20white%20counterparts.

36. Texas Maternal Mortality and Morbidity Review Committee and Texas Department of State Health Services, *Joint Biennial Report 2022*, updated October 2023, www.dshs.texas.gov/sites/default/files/legislative/2022-Reports/2022-MMMRC-DSHS-Joint-Biennial-Report.pdf.

37. Ariadna Huertas-Zurriaga et al., "Reproductive Decision-Making of Black Women Living with HIV: A Systematic Review," *Women's Health* 18 (2022), https://doi.org/10.1177/17455057221090827.

38. June Cross, dir., *Wilhemina's War*, Secret Daughter Productions, 2015.

39. Angela C. Incollingo Rodriguez et al, "Pregnant and Postpartum Women's Experiences of Weight Stigma in Healthcare," *BMC Pregnancy and Childbirth* 20 (2020): 1–10.

40. May Friedman, Carla Rice, and Emily R.M. Lind, "A High-Risk Body for Whom? On Fat, Risk, Recognition and Reclamation in

Restorying Reproductive Care through Digital Storytelling," *Feminist Encounters: A Journal of Critical Studies in Culture and Politics* 4, no. 2 (2020): 2.

41. Adriana Kohler, "Too Many Texas Mothers and Babies Are Dying. It's Time to Act," *Fort Worth Star-Telegram*, February 6, 2018, www.star-telegram.com/opinion/opn-columns-blogs/other-voices/article198661704.html.

42. Monica Saucedo et al., "Understanding Maternal Mortality in Women with Obesity and the Role of Care They Receive: A National Case-Control Study," *International Journal of Obesity* 45, no. 1 (2021): 258–65, https://doi.org/10.1038/s41366-020-00691-4.

43. Heather Frey et al., "Association of Prepregnancy Body Mass Index with Risk of Severe Maternal Morbidity and Mortality among Medicaid Beneficiaries," *JAMA Network Open* 5, no. 6 (2022): 1–14, https://doi.org/10.1001/jamanetworkopen.2022.18986.

44. Friedman, Rice, and Lind, "High-Risk Body for Whom?"

2. REPRODUCTIVE JUSTICE: AN AMERICAN GRAMMAR

1. Jo Yurcaba, "Law Professor Khiara Bridges Calls Sen. Josh Hawley's Questions about Pregnancy Transphobic," *NBC News*, July 13, 2022, www.nbcnews.com/nbc-out/out-politics-and-policy/law-professor-khiara-bridges-calls-sen-josh-hawleys-questions-pregnanc-rcna38015.

2. Hortense J. Spillers, "Mama's Baby, Papa's Maybe: An American Grammar Book," *Diacritics* 17, no. 2 (1987): 65.

3. Spillers, "Mama's Baby," 68.

4. Spillers, "Mama's Baby," 80.

5. Christina Sharpe, *In the Wake: On Blackness and Being* (Durham, NC: Duke University Press, 2016), 76.

6. Selamawit Terrefe, "What Exceeds the Hold? An Interview with Christina Sharpe," *Rhizomes* 29 (2016), www.rhizomes.net/issue29/terrefe.html.

7. Sharpe, "What Exceeds the Hold?," 75.

8. Cammy Pedroja, "Rep. Cori Bush Says 'Birthing People' in 'Maternal Health Crisis' Testimony, and Twitter Goes Nuts," *Newsweek*, October 3, 2021, www.newsweek.com/rep-cori-bush-says-birthing-people-maternal-health-crisis-testimony-twitter-goes-nuts-1589401.

9. Laer Streeter, "Reimagining Postpartum Care: A Call for Greater Inclusivity," American College of Obstetricians and Gynecologists, June 21, 2024, www.acog.org/news/news-articles/2024/06/reimagining-postpartum-care.

10. Eliza Sullivan, "Fat Is Not a Bad Word," *Teen Vogue*, July 22, 2021, www.teenvogue.com/story/fat-is-not-a-bad-word.

11. Saidiya Hartman, "Venus in Two Acts," *Small Axe: A Journal of Criticism* 12, no. 2 (2008): 11.

12. S.R. Toliver, *Recovering Black Storytelling in Qualitative Research: Endarkened Storywork* (New York: Routledge, 2022), xx.

13. adrienne maree brown, *Emergent Strategy: Shaping Change, Changing Worlds* (Chico, CA: AK Press, 2017).

14. Loretta J. Ross and Rickie Solinger, *Reproductive Justice: An Introduction* (Oakland: University of California Press, 2017), 209.

15. Marquis Bey, *Black Trans Feminism* (Durham, NC: Duke University Press, 2022), 3.

16. Kai M. Green, "The Essential I/Eye in We: A Black Transfeminist Approach to Ethnographic Film," *Black Camera: An International Film Journal*, n.s., 6, no. 2 (2015): 196, https://doi.org/10.2979/blackcamera.6.2.187.

17. "What Is Birth Justice?" Voices for Birth Justice, accessed June 19, 2022, https://voicesforbirthjustice.org/birth-justice/.

18. Joia Crear-Perry et al., "Social and Structural Determinants of Health Inequities in Maternal Health," *Journal of Women's Health* 30, no. 2 (2021): 230–35.

19. See Heidi L. Janz, "Ableism: The Undiagnosed Malady Afflicting Medicine," *Canadian Medical Association Journal* 191, no. 17 (2019): E478–E479, https://doi.org/10.1503/cmaj.180903.

20. Tien Sydnor-Campbell, "Sex, Sexuality, and the Disabled Black Woman," *Journal of Black Sexuality and Relationships* 3, no. 3 (2017): 72, https://dx.doi.org/10.1353/bsr.2017.0004.

21. May Friedman, Carla Rice, and Emily R.M. Lind. "A High-Risk Body for Whom? On Fat, Risk, Recognition and Reclamation in Restorying Reproductive Care through Digital Storytelling," *Feminist Encounters: A Journal of Critical Studies in Culture and Politics* 4, no. 2 (2020): 2, https://doi.org/10.20897/femenc/8524.

22. Cara Page, Erica Woodland, and Aurora Levins Morales, *Healing Justice Lineages: Dreaming at the Crossroads of Liberation, Collective Care, and Safety* (Berkeley, CA: North Atlantic Books, 2023), 57.

23. Saidiya Hartman, *Lose Your Mother: A Journey along the Atlantic Slave Route* (New York: Farrar, Straus, and Giroux, 2007), 6.

24. Yoshiko Iwai, Zahra H. Khan, and Sayantani DasGupta, "Abolition Medicine," *The Lancet* 396, no. 10245 (2020): 159, https://doi.org/10.1016/s0140-6736(20)31566-x.

3. REMEMORY: A REPRODUCTIVE JUSTICE MIXTAPE

1. See Brittney Cooper's "(Un)Clutching My Mother's Pearls, or Ratchetness and the Residue of Respectability," in *The Crunk Feminist Collection*, ed. Britney Cooper, Susana Morris, and Robin Boylorn (New York: Feminist Press at the City University of New York, 2017), 217–21.

2. Monica Simpson, "Now More Than Ever, We Need to Keep Trusting Black Women," *TheGrio*, June 28, 2023, https://thegrio.com/2023/06/28/now-more-than-ever-we-need-to-keep-trusting-black-women/.

3. Mary J. Blige, "My Life," *My Life*, MCA Records, 1994.

4. Tank and the Bangas, "Dope Girl Magic," *Green Balloon*, UMG Recordings, 2019.

5. Jhené Aiko, "Trigger Protection Mantra," Def Jam Recordings, 2019.

6. Toni Morrison, *Beloved* (New York: Alfred A. Knopf, 1987), 43.

7. Morrison, *Beloved*, 43.

8. Edwidge Danticat, *Breath, Eyes, Memory* (New York: Soho Press, 1994).

9. Michelle Browder, "The Official Guide to the Anarcha Lucy Betsey Third Annual Day of Reckoning Conference," Anarcha Lucy Betsey website, www.anarchalucybetsey.org/2024conference.

10. Brad Harper, "Artist Michelle Browder Fights for Accurate History in Alabama," *Montgomery Advertiser*, March 16, 2022, www.montgomeryadvertiser.com/in-depth/opinion/2022/03/13/michelle-browder-alabama-usa-today-women-of-the-year/6881444001/.

11. Browder v. Gayle, 142 F. Supp. 707 (Dist. Court, MD Alabama 1956).

12. Linda Matchan, "A Mother's Pain: Alabama's Gynecology Memorial Statue Sparks Debate," *Washington Post*, October 1, 2021, www.washingtonpost.com/entertainment/mothers-gynecology-alabama-memorial-statue/2021/10/01/cca0a788-21fd-11ec-8200-5e3fd4c49f5e_story.html.

13. Kriston Capps, "A Monument to the Enslaved 'Mothers of Gynecology' Rises in Montgomery," *Bloomberg*, May 10, 2022, www.bloomberg.com/news/articles/2022-05-10/forging-a-memorial-to-the-forgotten-mothers-of-gynecology.

14. Nikki Rojas, "How Lucy, Betsey, and Anarcha Became Foremothers of Gynecology," *Harvard Gazette*, March 30, 2023, https://news.harvard.edu/gazette/story/2023/03/how-lucy-betsey-and-anarcha-became-foremothers-of-gynecology/#:~:text=Anarcha%20endured%20at%20least%2030,to%20urinary%20incontinence%2C%20Marcelin%20noted.

15. Sarah Kuta, "Subjected to Painful Experiments and Forgotten, Enslaved 'Mothers of Gynecology' Are Honored with New Monument," *Smithsonian Magazine*, May 11, 2022, www.smithsonianmag.com/smart-news/mothers-of-gynecology-monument-honors-enslaved-women-180980064/.

16. Ntozake Shange, *for colored girls who have considered suicide, when the rainbow is enuf: a choreopoem* (New York: Scribner, 2022), 5.

17. Cheri Mossburg and Taylor Romine, "Widower of Black Woman Who Died Hours after Childbirth Files Civil Rights Lawsuit against Cedars-Sinai," *CNN*, May 6, 2022, www.cnn.com/2022/05/06/us/california-civil-rights-lawsuit-cedars-sinai/index.html.

18. Otis W. Brawley, "The Study of Untreated Syphilis in the Negro Male," *International Journal of Radiation Oncology Biology Physics* 40, no. 1 (1998): 5–8, https://doi.org/10.1016/s0360-3016(97)00835-3.

19. Fred de Sam Lazaro and Simeon Lancaster, "Alabama Artist Works to Correct Historical Narrative around Beginnings of Gynecology," *PBS News*, February 27, 2023, www.pbs.org/newshour/show/alabama-artist-works-to-correct-historical-narrative-around-beginnings-of-gynecology.

20. "Mothers of Gynecology for the Relf Sisters Fund," GoFundMe, accessed May 10, 2024, www.gofundme.com/f/the-relf-sisters-fund.

21. Bettina Judd, *patient: poems* (Pittsburgh, PA: Black Lawrence Press, 2014), 8.

22. Judd, *patient*, 75.

23. Amy Furr, "Video: Women 'Twerking for Abortions' in Dallas as SCOTUS Overrules *Roe v. Wade*," *Breitbart*, June 24, 2022, www.breitbart.com/politics/2022/06/24/video-women-twerking-abortions-dallas-scotus-overrules-roe-v-wade/.

24. adrienne maree brown, *Pleasure Activism: The Politics of Feeling Good* (Chico, CA: AK Press, 2019), 200.

25. Daphne Brooks, *Liner Notes for the Revolution: The Intellectual Life of Black Feminist Sound* (Cambridge, MA: Harvard University Press, 2023), 3.

26. See Cooper, "(Un)Clutching My Mother's Pearls"; L.H. Stallings, "Hip Hop and the Black Ratchet Imagination," *Palimpsest: A Journal on Women, Gender, and the Black International* 2, no. 2 (2013): 135–39, https://doi.org/10.1353/pal.2013.0026; and Bettina L. Love, "A Ratchet Lens: Black Queer Youth, Agency, Hip Hop, and the Black Ratchet Imagination," *Educational Researcher* 46, no. 9 (2017): 539–47, https://doi.org/10.3102/0013189x17736520.

27. Cooper, "(Un)Clutching My Mother's Pearls," 220.

28. Anastasia Tsioulcas and Chloe Veltman, "Tory Lanez Sentenced to 10 Years for Megan Thee Stallion Shooting," *NPR*,

August 9, 2023, www.npr.org/2023/08/08/1181702809/tory-lanez-megan-thee-stallion.

29. Rachel Treisman, Brakkton Booker, and Vanessa Romo, "Kentucky Grand Jury Indicts 1 of 3 Officers in Breonna Taylor Case," *NPR*, September 23, 2020, www.npr.org/sections/live-updates-protests-for-racial-justice/2020/09/23/914250463/breonna-taylor-charging-decision-to-be-announced-this-afternoon-lawyer-says.

30. Megan Thee Stallion, "Why I Speak Up for Black Women," *New York Times*, October 13, 2020, www.nytimes.com/2020/10/13/opinion/megan-thee-stallion-black-women.html.

31. reelaviolette botts-ward, *mourning my inner [black girl] child* (Oakland, CA: Nomadic Press, 2021), 104.

32. Audrey Lyndon et al., "Emotional Safety Is Patient Safety," *BMJ Quality and Safety* 32, no. 7 (2023): 369, https://doi.org/10.1136/bmjqs-2022-015573.

33. Lyndon et al., "Emotional Safety Is Patient Safety," 370.

34. botts-ward, *mourning my inner [black girl] child*, 100.

35. Lucille Clifton, "why some people be mad at me sometimes," in *The Collected Poems of Lucille Clifton* (Rochester, NY: BOA Press, 2012), 262.

36. Judd, *patient*, 10.

4. IMAGINING LIVABLE BLACK FUTURES

1. Quoted in Robin D. G. Kelley, *Freedom Dreams: The Black Radical Imagination* (New York: Beacon Press, 2003), xxvii.

2. Kelley, *Freedom Dreams*, xviii.

3. See S.R. Toliver, *Recovering Black Storytelling in Qualitative Research: Endarkened Storywork* (New York: Routledge, 2022).

4. Kelley, *Freedom Dreams*, xix–xx.

5. Audre Lorde, "Man Child: A Black Lesbian Feminist's Response," in *Zami; Sister Outsider; Undersong* (Mechanicsburg, PA: Quality Paperback Book Club, 1993), 72.

6. Lorde, "Man Child," 78.

7. Lorde, "Man Child," 74.

8. See Dani McClain, *We Live for the We: The Political Power of Black Motherhood* (Chico, CA: AK Press, 2019).

9. Ida B. Wells-Barnett, "Letter, Ida B. Wells to Daughters Ida and Alfreda, October 30, 1920," The Black Women's Suffrage Digital Collection, https://blackwomenssuffrage.dp.la/collections/ida-b-wells/ibwells-0008-009-09.

10. See Ida B. Wells-Barnett, *Crusade for Justice: The Autobiography of Ida B. Wells* (Chicago: University of Chicago Press, 1970), and Joy Davenport and Monica Land, dirs., *Fannie Lou Hamer's America*, Women Make Movies, 2023.

11. Octavia E. Butler, *Parable of the Sower* (New York: Grand Central Publishing, 2023).

12. adrienne maree brown, *Emergent Strategy: Shaping Change, Changing Worlds* (Chico, CA: AK Press, 2017), 3.

13. brown, *Emergent Strategy*, 6.

14. brown, *Emergent Strategy*, 17.

15. brown, *Emergent Strategy*, 18–19.

16. "Our Work," Full Frame Initiative, accessed November 7, 2024, www.fullframeinitiative.org/our-work/.

17. "Black Birthing Bill of Rights," National Association to Advance Black Birth, 2018, https://thenaabb.org/black-birthing-bill-of-rights/.

18. S.B. No. 8, Texas State Senate, May 13, 2021, https://capitol.texas.gov/tlodocs/87R/billtext/pdf/SB00008F.pdf.

19. Candice Norwood, "Policing and Surveillance: How Texas' Abortion Law Could Add to Systemic Racism," *The 19th*, September 14, 2021, https://19thnews.org/2021/09/texas-abortion-law-people-of-color/.

20. Melissa N. Montoya, Colleen Judge-Golden, and Jonas J. Swartz, "The Problems with Crisis Pregnancy Centers: Reviewing the Literature and Identifying New Directions for Future Research," *International Journal of Women's Health* 14 (2022): 757–63.

21. Dorothy E. Roberts, *Killing the Black Body: Race, Reproduction, and the Meaning of Liberty* (New York: Pantheon Books, 1997), 122–23.

22. Matt Lavietes, "Here's What Florida's 'Don't Say Gay' Bill Would Do and What It Wouldn't Do," *NBC News*, March 16, 2022, www.nbcnews.com/nbc-out/out-politics-and-policy/floridas-dont-say-gay-bill-actually-says-rcna19929.

23. Alex Nguyen and William Mehado, "Gov. Greg Abbott Signs Legislation Barring Trans Youth from Accessing Transition-Related Care," *Texas Tribune*, June 2, 2023, www.texastribune.org/2023/06/02/texas-gender-affirming-care-ban/.

24. See Audre Lorde, *A Burst of Light and Other Essays* (New York: Dover, 2017), 181.

25. Mariame Kaba, *We Do This 'til We Free Us: Abolitionist Organizing and Transforming Justice*, ed. Tamara K. Nopper (Chicago: Haymarket Press, 2021), 28.

26. Kaba, *We Do This*, 5.

5. ABOLITION MEDICINE

1. See Joshua M. Price, *Prison and Social Death* (New Brunswick, NJ: Rutgers University Press, 2015).

2. Yoshiko Iwai, Zahra H. Khan, and Sayantani DasGupta, "Abolition Medicine," *The Lancet* 396, no. 10245 (2020): 159.

3. Assata Shakur, *Assata: An Autobiography* (Chicago: Lawrence Hill Books, 2001), 130.

4. Damaris B. Hill, *A Bound Woman Is a Dangerous Thing: The Incarceration of African American Women from Harriet Tubman to Sandra Bland* (New York: Bloomsbury, 2019), 132.

5. See Stephen Dillon, "Possessed by Death: The Neoliberal-Carceral State, Black Feminism, and the Afterlife of Slavery," *Radical History Review* 112 (2012): 113–25.

6. Alys Eve Weinbaum, *The Afterlife of Reproductive Slavery: Biocapitalism and Black Feminism's Philosophy of History* (Durham, NC: Duke University Press, 2019), 2.

7. See Prison Policy Initiative's website at www.prisonpolicy.org/.

8. See Tien Sydnor-Campbell, "Sex, Sexuality, and the Disabled Black Woman," *Journal of Black Sexuality and Relationships* 3, no. 3 (2017): 65–79, https://dx.doi.org/10.1353/bsr.2017.0004.

9. Jacqueline Howard, "Beyoncé, Serena Williams Bring Attention to Risks of Childbirth for Black Women," *CNN*, August 6, 2018, https://edition.cnn.com/2018/08/06/health/beyonce-vogue-pregnancy-complication-bn/index.html.

10. Mariame Kaba, *We Do This 'til We Free Us: Abolitionist Organizing and Transforming Justice*, ed. Tamara K. Nopper (Chicago: Haymarket Press, 2021), 37.

11. This assertion is an adaptation and an update of Dorothy Roberts's illuminating point in *Killing the Black Body* that "every indignity that comes from the denial of reproductive autonomy can be found in slave women's lives." *Killing the Black Body: Race, Reproduction, and the Meaning of Liberty* (New York: Pantheon Books, 1997), 23.

12. See Dorothy E. Roberts, "Unshackling Black Motherhood," *Michigan Law Review* 95 (1996): 959, https://doi.org/10.2307/1290050.

13. Crystal M. Hayes, Carolyn Sufrin, and Jamila B. Perritt, "Reproductive Justice Disrupted: Mass Incarceration as a Driver of Reproductive Oppression," *American Journal of Public Health* 110, no. S1 (2020): S21, https://doi.org/10.2105/ajph.2019.305407.

14. See the website for the REBUILD project at Darkness Rising, https://darknessrisingproject.org/help-me-find-a-therapist/.

15. See Bench Ansfield, Rachel Herzing, and Dean Spade, "Abolition Infrastructures: A Conversation on Transformative Justice with Rachel Herzing and Dean Spade," *Radical History Review*, no. 147 (2023): 187–203, https://doi.org/10.1215/01636545-10637246.

16. See Andrea Freeman, "Unmothering Black Women: Formula Feeding as an Incident of Slavery," *Hastings Law Journal* 69 (2017): 1545–1606, https://papers.ssrn.com/sol3/papers.cfm?abstract_id=3236940.

17. Byllye Avery's notion of the "conspiracy of silence" that surrounds conversations about sexual and reproductive health and Dian Millon's assertion that silence is colonialism's strongest defense shed light on just how much oppression relies on our

silence. It keeps us not only from healing but also from resisting. See Byllye Avery, "Empowerment through Wellness," *Yale Journal of Law and Feminism* 4 (1991): 147–54, https://heinonline.org/HOL/LandingPage?handle=hein.journals/yjfem4&div=18&id=&page=, and Dian Millon, "Telling Secrets: Sex, Power and Narratives in Indian Residential School Histories," *Canadian Woman Studies* 20, no. 2 (2000): 92–104, https://cws.journals.yorku.ca/index.php/cws/article/view/7615.

18. Hill, *Bound Woman*.
19. Hill, *Bound Woman*, xix.
20. Shakur, *Assata*, 126.
21. Shakur, *Assata*, 127.
22. Shakur, *Assata*, 210.
23. Shakur, *Assata*, 144.
24. Shakur, *Assata*, 53.
25. Joanne Braxton, *Black Women Writing Autobiography: A Tradition within a Tradition* (Philadelphia: Temple University Press, 1989), 21.
26. Joy James, "The Womb of Western Theory: Trauma, Time Theft, and the Captive Maternal," *Carceral Notebooks* 12, no. 1 (2016): 255, https://sites.williams.edu/jjames/files/2019/05/WombofWesternTheory2016.pdf.
27. James, "Womb of Western Theory," 286.
28. See Crystal M. Hayes and Anu Manchikanti Gomez, "Alignment of Abolition Medicine with Reproductive Justice," *AMA Journal of Ethics* 24, no. 3 (2022): 188–93, https://doi.org/10.1001/amajethics.2022.188.
29. Mariame Kaba, *We Do This 'til We Free Us: Abolitionist Organizing and Transforming Justice*, ed. Tamara K. Nopper (Chicago: Haymarket Press. 2021), 23.
30. Kaba, *We Do This*, 5.
31. Nhi Tran, Aminta Kouyate, and Monica U. Hahn, "Why Professionalism Demands Abolition of Carceral Approaches to Patients' Nonadherence Behaviors," *AMA Journal of Ethics* 24, no. 3 (2022): 182, https://doi.org/10.1001/amajethics.2022.181.

32. See Amy N. Sweigart and Michael J. Matteucci, "Fever, Sacral Pain, and Pregnancy: An Incarcerated Uterus," *Western Journal of Emergency Medicine* 9, no. 4 (2008): 232–34.

33. Esther Kaner, "Abolition Medicine: Dismantling Carceral Logics in Healthcare," National Survivor User Network, December 15, 2021, www.nsun.org.uk/abolition-medicine-dismantling-carceral-logics-in-healthcare/.

34. Khiara Bridges, *Reproducing Race: An Ethnography of Pregnancy as a Site of Racialization* (Berkeley: University of California Press, 2011), 76.

35. See Mia Mingus, "Medical Industrial Complex Visual," with Cara Page and Patty Berne, *Leaving Evidence* (blog), February 6, 2015, https://leavingevidence.wordpress.com/2015/02/06/medical-industrial-complex-visual/.

36. See Tran, Kouyate, and Hahn, "Why Professionalism Demands Abolition."

37. Hayes and Gomez, "Alignment of Abolition Medicine," 190.

38. Kaner, "Abolition Medicine."

39. Notably, the Prison Policy Initiative has been committed to addressing this.

40. Donna L. Hoyert, "Maternal Mortality Rates in the United States, 2020," Centers for Disease Control and Prevention, February 23, 2022, www.cdc.gov/nchs/data/hestat/maternal-mortality/2020/maternal-mortality-rates-2020.htm.

41. Audre Lorde, "A Litany for Survival," in *The Collected Poems of Audre Lorde* (New York: W. W. Norton, 1997), 255.

42. Malika Saada Saar et al., *The Sexual Abuse to Prison Pipeline: The Girls' Story* (Washington, DC: Center on Poverty and Inequality, Georgetown Law, 2015), https://genderjusticeandopportunity.georgetown.edu/wp-content/uploads/2020/06/The-Sexual-Abuse-To-Prison-Pipeline-The-Girls%E2%80%99-Story.pdf.

43. Achille Mbembé, "Necropolitics," *Public Culture* 15 (2003): 11–40, https://doi.org/10.1215/08992363-15-1-11.

44. "Covid-19's Impact on People in Prison," Equal Justice Initiative, April 16, 2021, https://eji.org/news/covid-19s-impact-on-people-in-prison/.

45. It is important to note that one storyteller shared that prison is where some actually receive health care. Carolyn Sufrin's *Jailcare: Finding the Safety Net for Women behind Bars* (Oakland: University of California Press, 2017) explores this contradictory dynamic: some who are incarcerated were so thoroughly marginalized in society before imprisonment (whether because of houselessness, addiction, etc.) that they were previously afraid to seek or were denied health care.

46. The film *Belly of the Beast* also explores medical harm via the sterilization of incarcerated women. See *Belly of the Beast*, dir. Erika Cohn, Idlewild Films, 2021, www.bellyofthebeastfilm.com/.

47. Mary Enoch Elizabeth Baxter, "Ain't I a Woman," YouTube, October 29, 2020, www.youtube.com/watch?v=ivj9Jt_ONbQ.

48. Baxter, "Ain't I a Woman."

49. Nicole Fleetwood, *Marking Time: Art in the Age of Mass Incarceration* (Cambridge, MA: Harvard University Press, 2020), 46.

50. James, "Womb of Western Theory," 281.

51. Dobbs v. Jackson Women's Health Organization, *SCOTUS Blog*, 2021, www.scotusblog.com/case-files/cases/dobbs-v-jackson-womens-health-organization/.

6. POLICING BLACK BIRTH

1. Arline T. Geronimus et al., "'Weathering' and Age Patterns of Allostatic Load Scores among Blacks and Whites in the United States," *American Journal of Public Health* 96, no. 5 (May 2006): 826, https://doi.org/10.2105/AJPH.2004.060749.

2. Saidiya Hartman, *Lose Your Mother: A Journey along the Atlantic Slave Route* (New York: Farrar, Straus, and Giroux, 2007), 6.

3. Andrea Freeman, "Unmothering Black Women: Formula Feeding as an Incident of Slavery," *Hastings Law Journal* 69 (2017): 1545–1606, https://papers.ssrn.com/sol3/papers.cfm?abstract_id=3236940.

4. Michele Goodwin, *Policing the Womb: Invisible Women and the Criminalization of Motherhood* (Cambridge: Cambridge University Press, 2020), 11.

5. Dorothy Roberts, *Torn Apart: How the Child Welfare System Destroys Black Families—and How Abolition Can Build a Safer World* (New York: Basic Books, 2022), 27.

6. Dorothy Roberts, "What the History of Criminalizing Black Mothers Tells Us about the Post-*Roe* Legal Landscape," interview by Dahlia Lithwick, *Slate*, July 5, 2022, https://slate.com/news-and-politics/2022/07/roe-v-wade-abortion-criminalizing-black-motherhood-mississippi-dobbs.html.

7. Frank Edwards et al., "Medical Professional Reports and Child Welfare System Infant Investigations: An Analysis of National Child Abuse and Neglect Data System Data," *Health Equity* 7, no. 1 (2023): 659, https://doi.org/10.1089/heq.2023.0136.

8. Edwards et al., "Medical Professional Reports," 660.

9. Roni Caryn Rabin, "Black Pregnant Women Are Tested More Frequently for Drug Use, Study Suggests," *New York Times*, April 14, 2023, www.nytimes.com/2023/04/14/health/black-mothers-pregnancy-drug-testing.html?smtyp=cur&smid=tw-nytimes.

10. Rabin, "Black Pregnant Women."

11. Arielle Dreher, "Study Reveals Bias in Drug Testing Pregnant Patients," *Axios*, April 17, 2023, www.axios.com/2023/04/17/study-bias-drug-testing-pregnant-patients.

12. Dreher, "Study Reveals Bias."

13. Christina Sharpe, *In the Wake: On Blackness and Being* (Durham, NC: Duke University Press, 2016), 104.

14. See Harriet A. Washington, *Medical Apartheid: The Dark History of Medical Experimentation on Black Americans from Colonial Times to the Present* (New York: Knopf Doubleday, 2008).

15. Sabia Wade, *Birthing Liberation: How Reproductive Justice Can Set Us Free* (Chicago: Chicago Review Press, 2023), 38.

16. Elizabeth O'Brien and Miriam Rich, "Obstetric Violence in Historical Perspective," *The Lancet* 399 (2022): 2183, https://doi.org/10.1016/S0140-6736(22)01022-4.

17. Afiya Center, "Press Conference: NGAN & AFIYA Center," Facebook video, April 6, 2023, www.facebook.com/theafiyacenter/videos/1580065935835495.

18. Simon McCormack, host, "How the 'Child Welfare' System Destroys Black Families with Prof. Dorothy Roberts," Season 2, Episode 7 of *NYCLU: ACLU of New York* podcast, September 14, 2023, www.nyclu.org/podcast/s2-ep-7-how-the-child-welfare-system-destroys-black-families-with-prof-dorothy-roberts.

19. Kerry Breen, "Baby Taken from Texas Couple after Home Birth Will Be Returned by Dallas Court," *CBS News*, April 20, 2023, www.cbsnews.com/news/temecia-rodney-mila-jackson-returned-home-birth-jaundice-texas/; "Newborn Mila Jackson Heading Home to Her Family after Grueling 22 Day Saga," Afiya Center, press release, April 20, 2023, www.theafiyacenter.org/press-releases/2023/4/20/newborn-mila-jackson-heading-home-to-her-family-after-grueling-22-day-saga.

20. *A Thousand and One*, dir. A.V. Rockwell, Focus Features, Universal Pictures, 2023, 7:31.

21. *A Thousand and One*, 1:45.

22. *A Thousand and One*, 29:07.

23. *A Thousand and One*, 45:55.

24. *A Thousand and One*, 46:50.

25. *A Thousand and One*, 1:10:02.

26. *A Thousand and One*, 1:47:21.

27. Roberts, *Torn Apart*, 240.

28. Roberts, *Torn Apart*, 251.

29. *A Thousand and One*, 1:44:21.

30. *A Thousand and One*, 1:45:48.

EPILOGUE

1. Nap Ministry, "Rest Is Resistance," accessed June 19, 2022, https://thenapministry.com/.

2. Tricia Hersey, *Rest Is Resistance: A Manifesto* (New York: Little, Brown Spark, 2022).

3. Daphne Brooks, *Liner Notes for the Revolution: The Intellectual Life of Black Feminist Sound* (Cambridge, MA: Harvard University Press, 2023).

4. Bonnie Stabile, "High Noon for Reproductive Rights at the Supreme Court," *Ms. Magazine,* March 27, 2024, https://msmagazine.com/2024/03/27/mifepristone-supreme-court-abortion-pill-rally-demonstration/.

5. "Bans Off Our Bodies," Planned Parenthood, accessed January 5, 2023, www.plannedparenthoodaction.org/rightfully-ours/bans-off-our-bodies/about-bans-off-our-bodies.

6. Kendall, "What Are Crisis Pregnancy Centers?," *Planned Parenthood Blog,* November 4, 2021, www.plannedparenthood.org/blog/what-are-crisis-pregnancy-centers.

7. Valerie Gonza Lawsuit after Being Jailed on Murder Charge over Abortion Can Proceed, Judge Rules," Associated Press, July 24, 2024, https://apnews.com/article/texas-abortion-arrest-0a78cbb8f44cc24c3c9c811e1cc2b4d3.

8. Eleanor Klibanoff, "Texas Supreme Court Blocks Order Allowing Abortion; Woman Who Sought It Leaves State," *Texas Tribune,* December 11, 2023, www.texastribune.org/2023/12/11/texas-abortion-lawsuit-kate-cox/.

9. Mario Snipe, "The Black Reproductive Justice Leaders in a Post-Dobbs Era," *Capital B,* June 17, 2024, https://capitalbnews.org/post-dobbs-era-black-women/.

10. Kavitha Surana, "Abortion Bans Have Delayed Emergency Medical Care. In Georgia, Experts Say This Mother's Death Was Preventable," *ProPublica,* September 16, 2024, www.propublica.org/article/georgia-abortion-ban-amber-thurman-death.

11. Surana, "Abortion Bans."

12. Surana, "Abortion Bans."

13. Kavitha Surana, "Afraid to Seek Care amid Georgia's Abortion Ban, She Stayed at Home and Died," *ProPublica,* September 18, 2024, www.propublica.org/article/candi-miller-abortion-ban-death-georgia.

14. Surana, "Afraid to Seek Care."

15. Surana, "Afraid to Seek Care."

16. "Statement on the Deaths of Georgia Women Amber Thurman and Candi Miller," Feminist Women's Health Center,

press release, September 20, 2024, https://feministcenter.org/press/statement-on-the-deaths-of-georgia-women-amber-thurman-and-candi-miller/.

17. Assata Shakur, *Assata: An Autobiography* (Chicago: Lawrence Hill Books, 2001), 258.

18. Shakur, *Assata*, 259.

19. Cheryll Greene, "Word from a Sister in Exile," *Essence Magazine*, February 1988, 120.

20. Snipe, "Black Reproductive Justice Leaders."

21. Snipe, "Black Reproductive Justice Leaders."

BIBLIOGRAPHY

Aiko, Jhené. "Trigger Protection Mantra." Def Jam Recordings, 2019.
Altschuler, Glenn C. "Six Reasons Why Moms for Liberty Is an Extremist Organization." *The Hill*, July 9, 2023. https://thehill.com/opinion/education/4086179-six-reasons-why-moms-for-liberty-is-an-extremist-organization/.
Ani, Amanishakete. "C-Section and Racism: 'Cutting' to the Heart of the Issue for Black Women and Families." *Journal of African American Studies* 19 (2015): 343–61. https://doi.org/10.1007/s12111-015-9310-4.
Ansfield, Bench, Rachel Herzing, and Dean Spade. "Abolition Infrastructures: A Conversation on Transformative Justice with Rachel Herzing and Dean Spade." *Radical History Review*, no. 147 (2023): 187–203. https://doi.org/10.1215/01636545-10637246.
Avery, Byllye. "Empowerment through Wellness." *Yale Journal of Law and Feminism* 4 (1991): 147–54. https://heinonline.org/HOL/LandingPage?handle=hein.journals/yjfem4&div=18&id=&page=.
Baker, Brea. "This Black Family's Newborn Was Taken by CPS after Home Birth. It's Time for Reproductive Justice." *Refinery29*, April 13, 2023. www.refinery29.com/en-us/2023/04/11358435/baby-taken-by-cps-home-birth.

Barcelona, Veronica, Virginia Jenkins, Laura E. Britton, and Bethany G. Everett. "Adverse Pregnancy and Birth Outcomes in Sexual Minority Women from the National Survey of Family Growth." *BMC Pregnancy and Childbirth* 22, no. 1 (2022): 923. https://doi.org/10.1186/s12884-022-05271-0.

Baxter, Mary Enoch Elizabeth. "Ain't I a Woman." YouTube, October 29, 2020. www.youtube.com/watch?v=ivj9Jt_ONbQ.

Benjamin, Ruha. *Imagination: A Manifesto.* Norton Short. New York: W. W. Norton, 2024.

Bey, Marquis. *Black Trans Feminism.* Durham, NC: Duke University Press, 2022.

Blige, Mary J. "My Life." *My Life.* MCA Records, 1994.

Bosman, Julie. "After Water Fiasco, Trust in Officials Is in Short Supply in Flint." *New York Times*, October 8, 2016. www.nytimes.com/2016/10/09/us/after-water-fiasco-trust-of-officials-is-in-short-supply-in-flint.html.

botts-ward, reelaviolette. *mourning my inner [black girl] child.* Oakland, CA: Nomadic Press, 2021.

Brawley, Otis W. "The Study of Untreated Syphilis in the Negro Male." *International Journal of Radiation Oncology Biology Physics* 40, no. 1 (1998): 5–8. https://doi.org/10.1016/s0360-3016(97)00835-3.

Braxton, Joanne M. *Black Women Writing Autobiography: A Tradition within a Tradition.* Philadelphia: Temple University Press, 1989.

Breen, Kerry. "Baby Taken from Texas Couple after Home Birth Will Be Returned by Dallas Court." *CBS News*, April 20, 2023. www.cbsnews.com/news/temecia-rodney-mila-jackson-returned-home-birth-jaundice-texas/.

Bridges, Khiara. *Reproducing Race: An Ethnography of Pregnancy as a Site of Racialization.* Oakland: University of California Press, 2011.

Brookins, KB. "Sexting at the Gynecologist." *Poets Reading the News*, May 19, 2021. www.poetsreadingthenews.com/2021/05/sexting-at-the-gynecologist/.

Brookins, KB. "This Is What It's Like Going to the Gynecologist When You're Black, Trans and in Texas." *HuffPost*, February 10, 2022. www.huffpost.com/entry/black-trans-texas-abortion-gynecologist_n_61f7fe58e4b04f9a12c06a7a.

Brooks, Daphne. *Liner Notes for the Revolution: The Intellectual Life of Black Feminist Sound*. Cambridge, MA: Harvard University Press, 2023.

Browder, Michelle. "The Official Guide to the Anarcha Lucy Betsey Third Annual Day of Reckoning Conference." Anarcha Lucy Betsey website, 2024. www.anarchalucybetsey.org/2024conference.

brown, adrienne maree. *Emergent Strategy: Shaping Change, Changing Worlds*. Chico, CA: AK Press, 2017.

brown, adrienne maree. *Pleasure Activism: The Politics of Feeling Good*. Chico, CA: AK Press, 2019.

Butler, Octavia E. *Parable of the Sower*. New York: Grand Central Publishing, 2023.

Capps, Kriston. "A Monument to the Enslaved 'Mothers of Gynecology' Rises in Montgomery." *Bloomberg*, May 10, 2022. www.bloomberg.com/news/articles/2022-05-10/forging-a-memorial-to-the-forgotten-mothers-of-gynecology.

Clifton, Lucille. "why some people be mad at me sometimes." In *The Collected Poems of Lucille Clifton*, 262. Rochester, NY: BOA Press, 2012.

Cohn, Erika, dir. *Belly of the Beast*. Idlewild Films, 2021. www.bellyofthebeastfilm.com/.

Coleman, Kayden. "I'm a Transgender Dad. Here's What People Get Wrong about Me." *Yahoo!*, March 31, 2023. www.yahoo.com/news/m-transgender-dad-people-wrong-145309062.html?guccounter=1&guce_referrer=aHR0cHM6Ly93d3cuZ29vZ2xlLmNvbS8&guce_referrer_sig=AQAAAGB0CVTFdxFhD4s40FCwJWOghEybxf6Z98AGuPqzOOsmmv7iHcwQq9TqsOBLI3DlFbRxFmmlw7-eRDrD7Qw26J98MA9LE6ThHF5nQBYZ457R7ZJNnJb_OAuuiWjhpQljXEgi-EUtkNb05RAAgHyV2lYtpQfnxPewh-CloRsB3PPB.

Combahee River Collective. *The Combahee River Collective Statement* (1977). Reprinted as a reading on the Yale University, American Studies website. https://americanstudies.yale.edu/sites/default/files/files/Keyword%20Coalition_Readings.pdf.

Cooper, Brittney C. "(Un)clutching My Mother's Pearls, or Ratchetness and the Residue of Respectability." In *The Crunk Feminist Collection*, edited by Britney Cooper, Susana Morris, and Robin Boylorn, 217–21. New York: Feminist Press at the City University of New York, 2017.

Crear-Perry, Joia, Rosaly Correa-de-Araujo, Tamara Lewis Johnson, Monica R. McLemore, Elizabeth Neilson, and Maeve Wallace. "Social and Structural Determinants of Health Inequities in Maternal Health." *Journal of Women's Health* 30, no. 2 (2021): 230–35. https://doi.org/10.1089/jwh.2020.8882.

Cross, June, dir. *Wilhemina's War*. Secret Daughter Productions, 2015.

Crossley, Mary. "Reproducing Dignity: Race, Disability, and Reproductive Controls." *U.C. Davis Law Review* 54 (Spring 2020).

Cueto, Isabella, and Lacey Lyons. "Why Am I Having to Explain This? Seven Stories of Barriers to Reproductive Care for Those with Disabilities." *STAT*, November 8, 2023. www.statnews.com/2023/01/04/pregnancy-abortion-disability-health-chronic-disease/.

Danticat, Edwidge. *Breath, Eyes, Memory*. New York: Soho Press, 1994.

Davenport, Joy, and Monica Land, dirs. *Fannie Lou Hamer's America*. DVD. San Francisco: Women Make Movies, 2023.

Davis, Dána-Ain. *Reproductive Injustice: Racism, Pregnancy, and Premature Birth*. New York: New York University Press, 2019.

Dekker, Rebecca, host. "Black-Led Queer and Trans Birth Work with Mystique Hargrove, Kortney Lapeyrolerie, and Nadine Ashby." Episode 182 of *Evidence Based Birth* podcast. July 28, 2023. https://evidencebasedbirth.com/black-led-queer-and-trans-birth-work-with-mystique-hargrove-kortney-lapeyrolerie-and-nadine-ashby/.

de Sam Lazaro, Fred, and Simeon Lancaster. "Alabama Artist Works to Correct Historical Narrative around Beginnings of Gynecology." *PBS News*, February 27, 2023. www.pbs.org/newshour/show/alabama-artist-works-to-correct-historical-narrative-around-beginnings-of-gynecology.

Dillon, Stephen. "Possessed by Death: The Neoliberal-Carceral State, Black Feminism, and the Afterlife of Slavery." *Radical History Review* 112 (2012): 113–25. https://doi.org/10.1215/01636545-1416196.

Dirks, Sandhya. "Criminalization of Pregnancy Has Already Been Happening to the Poor and Women of Color." *NPR*, August 3, 2022. www.npr.org/2022/08/03/1114181472/criminalization-of-pregnancy-has-already-been-happening-to-the-poor-and-women-of.

Dreher, Arielle. "Study Reveals Bias in Drug Testing Pregnant Patients." *Axios*, April 17, 2023. www.axios.com/2023/04/17/study-bias-drug-testing-pregnant-patients.

Edwards, Frank, Sarah C.M. Roberts, Kathleen S. Kenny, Mical Raz, Matty Lichtenstein, and Mishka Terplan. "Medical Professional Reports and Child Welfare System Infant Investigations: An Analysis of National Child Abuse and Neglect Data System Data." *Health Equity* 7, no. 1 (2023): 653–62. https://doi.org/10.1089/heq.2023.0136.

Ehrenreich, Barbara, and Deirdre English. *Witches, Midwives, and Nurses: A History of Women Healers*. New York: Feminist Press at the City University of New York, 2010.

Equal Justice Initiative. "Covid-19's Impact on People in Prison." April 16, 2021. https://eji.org/news/covid-19s-impact-on-people-in-prison/.

Evans, Stephanie Y., Sarita K. Davis, Leslie R. Hinkson, and Deanna J. Wathington. "Introduction: Race, Gender, and Public Health: Social Justice and Wellness Work." In *Black Women and Public Health: Strategies to Name, Locate and Change Systems of Power*, edited by Stephanie Y. Evans, Sarita K. Davis, Leslie R. Hinkson, and Deanna J. Wathington, 1–32. Albany: State University of New York Press, 2022.

Evans-Winters, Venus E. *Black Feminism in Qualitative Inquiry: A Mosaic for Writing Our Daughter's Body*. London: Routledge, 2019.

Falu, Nessette. *Unseen Flesh: Gynecology and Black Queer Worth-Making in Brazil*. Durham, NC: Duke University Press. 2023.

Firth, Shannon. "Anti-gay Stigma Shortens Lives." *U.S. News and World Report*, February 19, 2014. www.usnews.com/news/articles/2014/02/19/research-anti-gay-stigma-shortens-lives.

Fleetwood, Nicole. *Marking Time: Art in the Age of Mass Incarceration*. Cambridge, MA: Harvard University Press, 2020.

Freeman, Andrea. "Unmothering Black Women: Formula Feeding as an Incident of Slavery." *Hastings Law Journal* 69 (2017): 1545–1606. https://papers.ssrn.com/sol3/papers.cfm?abstract_id=3236940.

Frey, Heather A., Robert Ashmead, Alyssa Farmer, Yoshie H. Kim, Cynthia Shellhaas, Reena Oza-Frank, Rebecca D. Jackson, Maged M. Costantine, and Courtney D. Lynch. "Association of Prepregnancy Body

Mass Index with Risk of Severe Maternal Morbidity and Mortality among Medicaid Beneficiaries." *JAMA Network Open* 5, no. 6 (2022): 1–14. https://doi.org/10.1001/jamanetworkopen.2022.18986.

Friedman, May, Carla Rice, and Emily R. M. Lind. "A High-Risk Body for Whom? On Fat, Risk, Recognition and Reclamation in Restorying Reproductive Care through Digital Storytelling." *Feminist Encounters: A Journal of Critical Studies in Culture and Politics* 4, no. 2 (2020): 1–12. https://doi.org/10.20897/femenc/8524.

Full Frame Initiative. "Our Work." Accessed November 7, 2024. www.fullframeinitiative.org/our-work/.

Furr, Amy. "VIDEO: Women 'Twerking for Abortions' in Dallas as SCOTUS Overrules *Roe v. Wade*." *Breitbart*, June 24, 2022. www.breitbart.com/politics/2022/06/24/video-women-twerking-abortions-dallas-scotus-overrules-roe-v-wade/.

Garcia-Hallett, Janet. *Invisible Mothers: Unseen yet Hypervisible after Incarceration*. Oakland: University of California Press, 2022.

Geronimus, Arline T. *Weathering: The Extraordinary Stress of Ordinary Life in an Unjust Society*. New York: Little, Brown Spark, 2023.

Geronimus, Arline T., Margaret Hicken, Danya Keene, and John Bound. "'Weathering' and Age Patterns of Allostatic Load Scores among Blacks and Whites in the United States." *American Journal of Public Health* 96, no. 5 (May 2006): 826–33. https://doi.org/10.2105/AJPH.2004.060749.

GoFundMe. "Mothers of Gynecology for the Relf Sisters Fund." Accessed May 10, 2024. www.gofundme.com/f/the-relf-sisters-fund.

Gonzalez, Valerie. "Texas Woman's Lawsuit after Being Jailed on Murder Charge over Abortion Can Proceed, Judge Rules." Associated Press, July 24, 2024. https://apnews.com/article/texas-abortion-arrest-0a78cbb8f44cc24c3c9c811e1cc2b4d3.

Goodwin, Michele. *Policing the Womb: Invisible Women and the Criminalization of Motherhood*. Cambridge: Cambridge University Press, 2020.

Green, Kai M. "The Essential I/Eye in We: A Black Transfeminist Approach to Ethnographic Film." *Black Camera: An International*

Film Journal, n.s., 6, no. 2 (2015): 187–200. https://doi.org/10.2979/blackcamera.6.2.187.

Green, Kai M., dir. *It Gets Messy in Here*. Film, 2011. Previously but not currently available on Vimeo. Recording in author's private collection.

Greene, Cheryll. "Word from a Sister in Exile." *Essence Magazine*, February 1988, 61–62, 120–22.

Guerrero, Maria. "Family of Transgender Woman Who Died in Dallas Police Custody Speak Out." *NBC 5 Dallas-Fort Worth*, June 13, 2022. www.nbcdfw.com/news/local/family-of-transgender-woman-who-died-in-dallas-police-custody-speak-out/2991447/.

Gumbs, Alexis Pauline. "Kakuya Collective: A Visionary Daughtering Webinar." *BrokenBeautiful Press*, November 2, 2016. https://brokenbeautiful.wordpress.com/2016/11/02/kakuya-collective-a-visionary-daughtering-webinar/.

Gumbs, Alexis Pauline, China Martens, and Mai'a Williams. *Revolutionary Mothering: Love on the Front Lines*. Oakland, CA: PM Press, 2016.

Hamer, Fannie Lou. "Nobody's Free until Everybody's Free: Speech Delivered at the Founding of the National Women's Political Caucus, Washington, DC, July 10, 1971." In *The Speeches of Fannie Lou Hamer: To Tell It Like It Is*, edited by Maegan Parker Brooks and Davis W. Houck, 134–39. Jackson: University Press of Mississippi, 2010.

Harper, Brad. "Artist Michelle Browder Fights for Accurate History in Alabama." *Montgomery Advertiser*, March 16, 2022. www.montgomeryadvertiser.com/in-depth/opinion/2022/03/13/michelle-browder-alabama-usa-today-women-of-the-year/6881444001/.

Hart, Ericka. "My Birthing Experience as a Black, Queer Parent Was Traumatic and—against All Odds—Joyful." *Refinery29*, April 13, 2013. www.refinery29.com/en-us/2023/04/11357620/ericka-hart-black-birthing-story-queer-parenting.

Hartman, Saidiya. *Lose Your Mother: A Journey along the Atlantic Slave Route*. New York: Farrar, Straus, and Giroux, 2007.

Hartman, Saidiya. "Venus in Two Acts." *Small Axe: A Journal of Criticism* 12, no. 2 (2008): 1–14. https://doi.org/10.1215/-12-2-1.

Hayes, Crystal M., and Anu Manchikanti Gomez. "Alignment of Abolition Medicine with Reproductive Justice." *AMA Journal of Ethics* 24, no. 3 (2022): 188–93. https://doi.org/10.1001/amajethics.2022.188.

Hayes, Crystal M., Carolyn Sufrin, and Jamila B. Perritt. "Reproductive Justice Disrupted: Mass Incarceration as a Driver of Reproductive Oppression." *American Journal of Public Health* 110, no. S1 (2020): S21–S24. https://doi.org/10.2105/ajph.2019.305407.

Hernandez, Joe. "Target Removes Some Pride Month Products after Threats against Employees. "*NPR*, May 24, 2023. www.npr.org/2023/05/24/1177963864/target-pride-month-lgbtq-products-threats.

Hersey, Tricia. *Rest Is Resistance: A Manifesto*. New York: Little, Brown Spark, 2022.

Hill, Damaris B. *A Bound Woman Is a Dangerous Thing: The Incarceration of African American Women from Harriet Tubman to Sandra Bland*. New York: Bloomsbury, 2019.

Hogarth, Rana A. *Medicalizing Blackness: Making Racial Difference in the Atlantic World, 1780–1840*. Chapel Hill: University of North Carolina Press, 2017.

Horner-Johnson, Willi, Mekhala Dissanayake, Nicole Marshall, and Jonathan M. Snowden. "Perinatal Health Risks and Outcomes among US Women with Self-Reported Disability, 2011–19: Study Examines Perinatal Health Risks and Outcomes among US Women with Self-Reported Disability." *Health Affairs* 41, no. 10 (2022): 1477–85. https://doi.org/10.1377/hlthaff.2022.00497.

Howard, Jacqueline. "Beyoncé, Serena Williams Bring Attention to Risks of Childbirth for Black Women." *CNN*, August 6, 2018. https://edition.cnn.com/2018/08/06/health/beyonce-vogue-pregnancy-complication-bn/index.html.

Hoyert, Donna L. "Maternal Mortality Rates in the United States, 2020." Centers for Disease Control and Prevention, February 23, 2022. www.cdc.gov/nchs/data/hestat/maternal-mortality/2020/maternal-mortality-rates-2020.htm.

Huertas-Zurriaga, Ariadna, Patrick A. Palmieri, Mariela P. Aguayo-Gonzalez, Karen A. Dominguez-Cancino, Cristina Casanovas-Cuellar,

Kara L. Vander Linden, Sandra K. Cesario, Joan E. Edwards, and Juan M. Leyva-Moral. "Reproductive Decision-Making of Black Women Living with HIV: A Systematic Review." *Women's Health* 18 (2022). https://doi.org/10.1177/17455057221090827.

Incollingo Rodriguez, Angela C., Stephanie M. Smieszek, Kathryn E. Nippert, and A. Janet Tomiyama. "Pregnant and Postpartum Women's Experiences of Weight Stigma in Healthcare." *BMC Pregnancy and Childbirth* 20 (2020): 1–10. https://doi.org/10.1186/s12884-020-03202-5.

Iwai, Yoshiko, Zahra H. Khan, and Sayantani DasGupta. "Abolition Medicine." *The Lancet* 396, no. 10245 (2020): 158–59. https://doi.org/10.1016/s0140-6736(20)31566-x.

Jain, Sagaree. "Two-Eyed Seeing: Decolonizing Methodologies for Reproductive Justice." *AMPLIFY*, May 19, 2020. https://medium.com/amplify/two-eyed-seeing-decolonizing-methodologies-for-reproductive-justice-ca16578e9e4a.

James, Joy. "The Womb of Western Theory: Trauma, Time Theft, and the Captive Maternal." *Carceral Notebooks* 12, no. 1 (2016): 253–96. https://sites.williams.edu/jjames/files/2019/05/WombofWesternTheory2016.pdf.

Janz, Heidi L. "Ableism: The Undiagnosed Malady Afflicting Medicine." *Canadian Medical Association Journal* 191, no. 17 (2019): E478–E479. https://doi.org/10.1503/cmaj.180903.

Judd, Bettina. *patient: poems*. Pittsburgh, PA: Black Lawrence Press, 2014.

Kaba, Mariame. *We Do This 'til We Free Us: Abolitionist Organizing and Transforming Justice*. Edited by Tamara K. Nopper. Chicago: Haymarket Press, 2021.

Kaner, Esther. "Abolition Medicine: Dismantling Carceral Logics in Healthcare." National Survivor User Network, December 15, 2021. www.nsun.org.uk/abolition-medicine-dismantling-carceral-logics-in-healthcare/.

Kapsalis, Terri. *Public Privates: Performing Gynecology from Both Ends of the Speculum*. Durham, NC: Duke University Press, 1997.

Karimi, Faith, and Natalie Johnson. "A Woman Left the ER to Find Another Hospital after a Long Wait. Two Hours Later, She Was Dead."

CNN, January 17, 2020. www.cnn.com/2020/01/17/us/tashonna-ward-death-questions-trnd/index.html.

Kelley, Robin D. G. *Freedom Dreams: The Black Radical Imagination*. New York: Beacon Press, 2003.

Kendall. "What Are Crisis Pregnancy Centers?" *Planned Parenthood Blog*, November 4, 2021. www.plannedparenthood.org/blog/what-are-crisis-pregnancy-centers.

King, Martin Luther. "Letter from Birmingham Jail." *Atlantic Monthly* [published under the title "The Negro Is Your Brother"], August 1963, 78–88. www.csuchico.edu/iege/_assets/documents/susi-letter-from-birmingham-jail.pdf.

King, Shantrice, host. "Decolonizing Healthcare." Season 5, Episode 1 of *Welcome to the (AfAm) House Podcast*. November 2021. https://open.spotify.com/episode/4Bgxwsw9zm81m5zR4eMqVY.

Klibanoff, Eleanor. "Texas Supreme Court Blocks Order Allowing Abortion; Woman Who Sought It Leaves State." *Texas Tribune*, December 11, 2023. www.texastribune.org/2023/12/11/texas-abortion-lawsuit-kate-cox/.

Kohler, Adriana. "Too Many Texas Mothers and Babies Are Dying. It's Time to Act." *Fort Worth Star-Telegram*, February 6, 2018. www.star-telegram.com/opinion/opn-columns-blogs/other-voices/article198661704.html.

Kuta, Sarah. "Subjected to Painful Experiments and Forgotten, Enslaved 'Mothers of Gynecology' Are Honored with New Monument." *Smithsonian Magazine*, May 11, 2022. www.smithsonianmag.com/smart-news/mothers-of-gynecology-monument-honors-enslaved-women-180980064/.

Lapid, Nancy. "U.S. Maternal Mortality More Than Doubled since 1999, Most Deaths among Black Women, Study Says." Reuters, July 3, 2023. www.reuters.com/world/us/us-maternal-mortality-more-than-doubled-since-1999-most-deaths-among-black-women-2023-07-03/.

Lavietes, Matt. "Here's What Florida's 'Don't Say Gay' Bill Would Do and What It Wouldn't Do." *NBC News*, March 16, 2022. www.nbcnews.com/nbc-out/out-politics-and-policy/floridas-dont-say-gay-bill-actually-says-rcna19929.

Lavietes, Matt. "Over Half of 2022's Most Challenged Books Have LGBTQ Themes." *NBC News*, April 25, 2023. www.nbcnews.com/nbc-out/out-politics-and-policy/half-2022s-challenged-books-lgbtq-themes-rcna81324.

Lindsey, Treva B. *America, Goddam: Violence, Black Women, and the Struggle for Justice*. Oakland: University of California Press, 2023.

Lithwick, Dahlia. "SCOTUS Wraps, Precedent Collapses, and KBJ Takes Her Oath." *Slate*, July 2022. https://slate.com/podcasts/amicus/2022/07/the-end-of-a-supreme-court-term-that-fundamentally-rearranged-rights.

Lorde, Audre. *A Burst of Light and Other Essays*. New York: Dover, 2017.

Lorde, Audre. "A Litany for Survival." In *The Collected Poems of Audre Lorde*, 215. New York: W. W. Norton, 1997.

Lorde, Audre. "Man Child: A Black Lesbian Feminist's Response." In *Zami; Sister Outsider; Undersong*, 72–80. Mechanicsburg, PA: Quality Paperback Book Club, 1993.

Lorde, Audre. "The Master's Tools Will Never Dismantle the Master's House." In *Zami; Sister Outsider; Undersong*, 110–13. Mechanicsburg, PA: Quality Paperback Book Club, 1993.

Lorde, Audre. *Zami; Sister Outsider; Undersong*. Mechanicsburg, PA: Quality Paperback Book Club, 1993.

Love, Bettina L. "A Ratchet Lens: Black Queer Youth, Agency, Hip Hop, and the Black Ratchet Imagination." *Educational Researcher* 46, no. 9 (2017): 539–47. https://doi.org/10.3102/0013189x17736520.

Lugones, Maria. "The Coloniality of Gender." In *The Palgrave Handbook of Gender and Development*, edited by Wendy Harcourt, 13–33. London: Palgrave Macmillan, 2016.

Lyndon, Audrey, Dána-Ain Davis, Anjana E. Sharma, and Karen A. Scott. "Emotional Safety Is Patient Safety." *BMJ Quality and Safety* 32, no. 7 (2023): 369–72. https://doi.org/10.1136/bmjqs-2022-015573.

Matchan, Linda. "A Mother's Pain: Alabama's Gynecology Memorial Statue Sparks Debate." *Washington Post*, October 1, 2021. www.washingtonpost.com/entertainment/mothers-gynecology-alabama-memorial-statue/2021/10/01/cca0a788-21fd-11ec-8200-5e3fd4c49f5e_story.html.

Mbembé, Achille. "Necropolitics." *Public Culture* 15 (2003): 11–40. https://doi.org/10.1215/08992363-15-1-11.

McClain, Dani. *We Live for the We: The Political Power of Black Motherhood.* Chico, CA: AK Press, 2019.

McCormack, Simon, host. "How the 'Child Welfare' System Destroys Black Families with Prof. Dorothy Roberts." Season 2, Episode 7 of *NYCLU: ACLU of New York* podcast. September 14, 2023. www.nyclu.org/podcast/s2-ep-7-how-the-child-welfare-system-destroys-black-families-with-prof-dorothy-roberts.

McLemore, Monica R., and Esther K. Choo. "The Right Decisions Need the Right Voices." *The Lancet* 394, no. 10204 (2019): 1113–1204. https://doi.org/10.1016/s0140-6736(19)32167-1.

Megan Thee Stallion. "Plan B." 1501 Certified Entertainment/300 Entertainment, 2022.

Megan Thee Stallion. "Why I Speak Up for Black Women." *New York Times*, October 13, 2020. www.nytimes.com/2020/10/13/opinion/megan-thee-stallion-black-women.html.

Million, Dian. "Telling Secrets: Sex, Power and Narratives in Indian Residential School Histories." *Canadian Woman Studies* 20, no. 2 (2000): 92–104. https://cws.journals.yorku.ca/index.php/cws/article/view/7615.

Mingus, Mia. "Medical Industrial Complex Visual." With Cara Page and Patty Berne. *Leaving Evidence* (blog), February 6, 2015. https://leavingevidence.wordpress.com/2015/02/06/medical-industrial-complex-visual/.

Mirza, Shabab Ahmed, and Caitlin Rooney. "Discrimination Prevents LGBTQ People from Accessing Health Care." Center for American Progress, August 23, 2022. www.americanprogress.org/article/discrimination-prevents-lgbtq-people-accessing-health-care/.

Montoya, Melissa N., Colleen Judge-Golden, and Jonas J. Swartz. "The Problems with Crisis Pregnancy Centers: Reviewing the Literature and Identifying New Directions for Future Research." *International Journal of Women's Health* 14 (2022): 757–63.

Morrison, Toni. *Beloved.* New York: Alfred A. Knopf, 1987.

Morrison, Toni. *The Bluest Eye.* New York: Plume, 1994.

Morrison, Toni. "The Site of Memory." In *Inventing the Truth: The Art and Craft of Memoir*, edited by William Zinsser, 85–102. New York: Houghton Mifflin, 1995.

Mossburg, Cheri, and Taylor Romine. "Widower of Black Woman Who Died Hours after Childbirth Files Civil Rights Lawsuit against Cedars-Sinai." *CNN*, May 6, 2022. www.cnn.com/2022/05/06/us/california-civil-rights-lawsuit-cedars-sinai/ind.

Nap Ministry. "Rest Is Resistance." Accessed June 19, 2022. https://thenapministry.com/.

Nash, Jennifer. *Birthing Black Mothers*. Durham, NC: Duke University Press, 2021.

National Association to Advance Black Birth. "Black Birthing Bill of Rights." 2018. https://thenaabb.org/black-birthing-bill-of-rights/.

NBC News. "Katrina Victims Blame Racism for Slow Aid." December 6, 2005. www.nbcnews.com/id/wbna10354221.

Nesbeth, Carlos, Kandala Rajiv, Sayed Najeeb, Ruksana Nazneen, and Banglore Murthy. "HIV Mortality Difference between Black and White Women." *Journal of Health Disparities Research and Practice* 11, no. 1 (2018): 179–90. https://digitalscholarship.unlv.edu/cgi/viewcontent.cgi?article=1699&context=jhdrp#:~:text=In%20these%20descriptive%20data%20from,that%20of%20their%20white%20counterparts.

Nguyen, Alex, and William Mehado. "Gov. Greg Abbott Signs Legislation Barring Trans Youth from Accessing Transition-Related Care." *Texas Tribune*, June 2, 2023. www.texastribune.org/2023/06/02/texas-gender-affirming-care-ban/.

Norwood, Candice. "Policing and Surveillance: How Texas' Abortion Law Could Add to Systemic Racism." *The 19th*, September 14, 2021. https://19thnews.org/2021/09/texas-abortion-law-people-of-color/.

O'Brien, Elizabeth, and Miriam Rich. "Obstetric Violence in Historical Perspective." *The Lancet* 399 (2022): 2183–85. https://doi.org/10.1016/S0140-6736(22)01022-4.

Owens, Deirdre Cooper. *Medical Bondage: Race, Gender, and the Origins of American Gynecology*. Albany: University of Georgia Press, 2017.

Page, Cara, Erica Woodland, and Aurora Levins Morales. *Healing Justice Lineages: Dreaming at the Crossroads of Liberation, Collective Care, and Safety*. Berkeley, CA: North Atlantic Books, 2023.

PBS. "Fannie Lou Hamer." Accessed March 10, 2024. www.pbs.org/wgbh/americanexperience/features/freedomsummer-hamer/.

Pedroja, Cammy. "Rep. Cori Bush Says 'Birthing People' in 'Maternal Health Crisis' Testimony, and Twitter Goes Nuts." *Newsweek*, October 3, 2021. www.newsweek.com/rep-cori-bush-says-birthing-people-maternal-health-crisis-testimony-twitter-goes-nuts-1589401.

Perkins-Valdez, Dolen. *Take My Hand*. New York: Penguin, 2022.

Pickens, Therí. "'You're Supposed to Be a Tall, Handsome, Fully Grown White Man': Theorizing Race, Gender, and Disability in Octavia Butler's *Fledgling*." *Journal of Literary and Cultural Disability Studies* 8, no. 1 (2014): 33–48. https://doi.org/10.3828/jlcds.2014.3.

Pillion, Dennis. "Monument to Mothers of Gynecology." *AL.com*, September 27, 2021. www.al.com/news/2021/09/monument-to-mothers-of-gynecology-unveiled-in-montgomery.html.

Planned Parenthood. "Bans Off Our Bodies." Accessed January 5, 2023. www.plannedparenthoodaction.org/rightfully-ours/bans-off-our-bodies/about-bans-off-our-bodies.

Price, Joshua M. *Prison and Social Death*. New Brunswick, NJ: Rutgers University Press, 2015.

Purdie-Vaughns, Valerie, and Richard P. Eibach. "Intersectional Invisibility: The Distinctive Advantages and Disadvantages of Multiple Subordinate-Group Identities." *Sex Roles* 59 (2008): 377–91. https://doi.org/10.1007/s11199-008-9424-4.

Purdy, Eve. "Embracing Messiness in Medicine, Research, and Ourselves." *ICE Blog: International Clinician Educators*, January 22, 2019. https://icenet.blog/2019/01/22/embracing-messiness-in-medicine-research-and-ourselves/.

Rabin, Roni Caryn. "Black Pregnant Women Are Tested More Frequently for Drug Use, Study Suggests." *New York Times*, April 14, 2023. www.nytimes.com/2023/04/14/health/black-mothers-pregnancy-drug-testing.html?smtyp=cur&smid=tw-nytimes.

Roberts, Dorothy E. *Killing the Black Body: Race, Reproduction, and the Meaning of Liberty*. New York: Pantheon Books, 1997.

Roberts, Dorothy. *Torn Apart: How the Child Welfare System Destroys Black Families—and How Abolition Can Build a Safer World*. New York: Basic Books, 2022.

Roberts, Dorothy E. "Unshackling Black Motherhood." *Michigan Law Review* 95 (1996): 938–64. https://doi.org/10.2307/1290050.

Roberts, Dorothy E. "What the History of Criminalizing Black Mothers Tells Us about the Post-*Roe* Legal Landscape." Interview by Dahlia Lithwick. *Slate*, July 5, 2022. https://slate.com/news-and-politics/2022/07/roe-v-wade-abortion-criminalizing-black-motherhood-mississippi-dobbs.html.

Rockwell, A. V., dir. *A Thousand and One*. Focus Features, Universal Pictures, 2023.

Rodriguez, Marcela. "Gov. Abbott Signs DEI Bill into Law, Dismantling Diversity Offices at Colleges." *Dallas Morning News*, June 14, 2023. www.dallasnews.com/news/education/2023/06/14/gov-abbott-signs-dei-bill-into-law-dismantling-diversity-offices-at-colleges/.

Rojas, Nikki. "How Lucy, Betsey, and Anarcha Became Foremothers of Gynecology." *Harvard Gazette*, March 30, 2023. https://news.harvard.edu/gazette/story/2023/03/how-lucy-betsey-and-anarcha-became-foremothers-of-gynecology/#:~:text=Anarcha%20endured%20at%20least%2030,to%20urinary%20incontinence%2C%20Marcelin%20noted.

Ross, Loretta J. "Conceptualizing Reproductive Justice Theory: A Manifesto for Activism." In *Radical Reproductive Justice: Foundation, Theory, Practice, Critique*, edited by Loretta J. Ross, Lynn Roberts, Erika Derkas, Whitney Peoples, and Pamela Bridgewater Toure, 170–232. New York: Feminist Press, 2017.

Ross, Loretta J. "Trust Black Women: Reproductive Justice and Eugenics." In *Radical Reproductive Justice: Foundation, Theory, Practice, Critique*, edited by Loretta J. Ross, Lynn Roberts, Erika Derkas, Whitney Peoples, and Pamela Bridgewater Toure, 58–85. New York: Feminist Press, 2017.

Ross, Loretta J., and Rickie Solinger. *Reproductive Justice: An Introduction*. Oakland: University of California Press, 2017.

Saar, Malika Saada, Rebecca Epstein, Lindsay Rosenthal, and Yasmin Vafa. *The Sexual Abuse to Prison Pipeline: The Girls' Story*. Washington, DC: Center on Poverty and Inequality, Georgetown Law, June 2020. https://genderjusticeandopportunity.georgetown.edu/wp-content/uploads/2020/06/The-Sexual-Abuse-To-Prison-Pipeline-The-Girls%E2%80%99-Story.pdf.

Saucedo, Monica, Ana Paula Esteves-Pereira, Lucile Pencolé, Agnès Rigouzzo, Alain Proust, Marie-Hélène Bouvier-Colle, and Catherine Deneux-Tharaux. "Understanding Maternal Mortality in Women with Obesity and the Role of Care They Receive: A National Case-Control Study." *International Journal of Obesity* 45, no. 1 (2021): 258–65. https://doi.org/10.1038/s41366-020-00691-4.

Scott, Karen A., Laura Britton, and Monica R. McLemore. "The Ethics of Perinatal Care for Black Women: Dismantling the Structural Racism in 'Mother Blame' Narratives." *Journal of Perinatal and Neonatal Nursing* 33, no. 2 (2019): 108–15. https://doi.org/10.1097/jpn.0000000000000394.

Shakur, Assata. *Assata: An Autobiography*. Chicago: Lawrence Hill Books, 2001.

Shange, Ntozake. *for colored girls who have considered suicide, when the rainbow is enuf: a choreopoem*. New York: Scribner, 2022.

Sharpe, Christina. *In the Wake: On Blackness and Being*. Durham, NC: Duke University Press, 2016.

Simpson, Monica. "Now More than Ever, We Need to Keep Trusting Black Women." *TheGrio*, June 28, 2023. https://thegrio.com/2023/06/28/now-more-than-ever-we-need-to-keep-trusting-black-women/.

SisterSong. "Reproductive Justice." Accessed March 10, 2023. www.sistersong.net/reproductive-justice.

Snipe, Mario. "The Black Reproductive Justice Leaders in a Post-Dobbs Era." *Capital B*, June 17, 2024. https://capitalbnews.org/post-dobbs-era-black-women/.

Solinger, Rickie, Madeline Fox, and Kayhan Irani. *Telling Stories to Change the World: Global Voices on the Power of Narrative to*

Build Community and Make Social Justice Claims. London: Routledge, 2008.

Southern Poverty Law Center. "Mississippi City's Water Problems Stem from Generations of Neglect." June 28, 2023. www.splcenter.org/news/2023/06/28/timeline-jackson-mississippi-water-problems#:~:text=Mississippi%20city's%20water%20problems%20stem%20from%20generations%20of%20neglect&text=On%20Aug.,no%20water%20service%20at%20all.

Spillers, Hortense J. "Mama's Baby, Papa's Maybe: An American Grammar Book." *Diacritics* 17, no. 2 (1987): 65–81.

Spivak, Gayatri Chakravorty. "Can the Subaltern Speak?" In *Marxism and the Interpretation of Culture*, edited by Cary Nelson and Lawrence Grossberg, 271–313. Champaign-Urbana: University of Illinois Press, 1988.

Stabile, Bonnie. "High Noon for Reproductive Rights at the Supreme Court." *Ms. Magazine*, March 27, 2024. https://msmagazine.com/2024/03/27/mifepristone-supreme-court-abortion-pill-rally-demonstration/.

Stallings, L. H. "Hip Hop and the Black Ratchet Imagination." *Palimpsest: A Journal on Women, Gender, and the Black International* 2, no. 2 (2013): 135–39. https://doi.org/10.1353/pal.2013.0026.

Streeter, Laer. "Reimagining Postpartum Care: A Call for Greater Inclusivity." American College of Obstetricians and Gynecologists, June 21, 2024. www.acog.org/news/news-articles/2024/06/reimagining-postpartum-care.

Strings, Sabrina. *Fearing the Black Body: The Racial Origins of Fat Phobia*. New York: New York University Press, 2019.

Sturgis, Sue. "Is a Duke Energy Power Plant Making Nearby Residents Sick?" *Facing South*, May 1, 2014. www.facingsouth.org/2014/05/is-a-duke-energy-power-plant-making-nearby-residen.html.

Sufrin, Carolyn. *Jailcare: Finding the Safety Net for Women behind Bars*. Oakland: University of California Press, 2017.

Sullivan, Eliza. "Fat Is Not a Bad Word." *Teen Vogue*, July 22, 2021. www.teenvogue.com/story/fat-is-not-a-bad-word.

Surana, Kavitha. "Abortion Bans Have Delayed Emergency Medical Care. In Georgia, Experts Say This Mother's Death Was Preventable."

ProPublica, September 16, 2024. www.propublica.org/article/georgia-abortion-ban-amber-thurman-death.

Surana, Kavitha. "Afraid to Seek Care amid Georgia's Abortion Ban, She Stayed at Home and Died." *ProPublica*, September 18, 2024. www.propublica.org/article/candi-miller-abortion-ban-death-georgia.

Sweigart, Amy N., and Michael J. Matteucci. "Fever, Sacral Pain, and Pregnancy: An Incarcerated Uterus." *Western Journal of Emergency Medicine* 9, no. 4 (2008): 232–34.

Sydnor-Campbell, Tien. "Sex, Sexuality, and the Disabled Black Woman." *Journal of Black Sexuality and Relationships* 3, no. 3 (2017): 65–79. https://dx.doi.org/10.1353/bsr.2017.0004.

Tagbo, Marie. "Sheryl Lee Ralph Releases Film 'Unexpected' on Hulu for World AIDS Day, Documenting the Stories of Black Women Living with HIV." GLAAD, December 1, 2023. https://glaad.org/sheryl-lee-ralph-releases-film-unexpected-on-hulu-for-world-aids-day-documenting-the-stories-of-black-women-living-with-hiv/.

Tank and the Bangas. "Dope Girl Magic." *Green Balloon*. UMG Recordings, 2019.

Terrefe, Selamawit. "What Exceeds the Hold? An Interview with Christina Sharpe." *Rhizomes* 29 (2016). www.rhizomes.net/issue29/terrefe.html.

Texas Maternal Mortality and Morbidity Review Committee and Texas Department of State Health Services. *Joint Biennial Report 2022*. Updated October 2023. www.dshs.texas.gov/sites/default/files/legislative/2022-Reports/2022-MMMRC-DSHS-Joint-Biennial-Report.pdf.

Thakur, Monika, Suzanne M. Jenkins, and Kunal Mahajan. "Cervical Insufficiency." StatPearls, National Library of Medicine, October 6, 2024. www.ncbi.nlm.nih.gov/books/NBK525954/.

Toliver, S.R. *Recovering Black Storytelling in Qualitative Research: Endarkened Storywork*. New York: Routledge, 2022.

Tran, Nhi, Aminta Kouyate, and Monica U. Hahn. "Why Professionalism Demands Abolition of Carceral Approaches to Patients' Nonadherence Behaviors." *AMA Journal of Ethics* 24, no. 3 (2022): 181–87. https://doi.org/10.1001/amajethics.2022.181.

Treisman, Rachel, Brakkton Booker, and Vanessa Romo. "Kentucky Grand Jury Indicts 1 of 3 Officers in Breonna Taylor Case." *NPR*, September 23, 2020. www.npr.org/sections/live-updates-protests-for-racial-justice/2020/09/23/914250463/breonna-taylor-charging-decision-to-be-announced-this-afternoon-lawyer-says.

Tsioulcas, Anastasia, and Chloe Veltman. "Tory Lanez Sentenced to 10 Years for Megan Thee Stallion Shooting." *NPR*, August 9, 2023. www.npr.org/2023/08/08/1181702809/tory-lanez-megan-thee-stallion.

Villarosa, Linda. "The Long Shadow of Eugenics in America." *New York Times Magazine*, June 8, 2022. www.nytimes.com/2022/06/08/magazine/eugenics-movement-america.html.

Villarosa, Linda. *Under the Skin: The Hidden Toll of Racism on American Lives and on the Health of Our Nation*. New York: Knopf Doubleday, 2022.

Voices for Birth Justice. "What Is Birth Justice?" Accessed June 19, 2022. https://voicesforbirthjustice.org/birth-justice/.

Wade, Sabia. *Birthing Liberation: How Reproductive Justice Can Set Us Free*. Chicago: Chicago Review Press, 2023.

Washington, Harriet A. *Medical Apartheid: The Dark History of Medical Experimentation on Black Americans from Colonial Times to the Present*. New York: Knopf Doubleday, 2008.

Weinbaum, Alys Eve. *The Afterlife of Reproductive Slavery: Biocapitalism and Black Feminism's Philosophy of History*. Durham, NC: Duke University Press, 2019.

Welch, Leseliey, Renee Branch Canady, Chelsea Harmell, Nicole White, and Lisa Kane Low. "We Are Not Asking Permission to Save Our Own Lives: Black-Led Birth Centers to Address Health Inequities." *Journal of Perinatal and Neonatal Nursing* 36, no. 2 (2022): 138–49. https://doi.org/10.1097/jpn.0000000000000649.

Wells-Barnett, Ida B. *Crusade for Justice: The Autobiography of Ida B. Wells*. Chicago: University of Chicago Press, 1970.

Wells-Barnett, Ida B. "Letter, Ida B. Wells to Daughters Ida and Alfreda, October 30, 1920." Black Women's Suffrage Digital Collection. https://blackwomenssuffrage.dp.la/collections/ida-b-wells/ibwells-0008-009-09.

WFAA Staff. "No Indictment in Case of Dallas Woman Who Died after Being Restrained by Police." *WFAA*, May 12, 2023. www.wfaa.com/article/news/local/dee-dee-hall-death-dallas-texas-investigation-police-grand-jury-indictment/287-8c9a35c4-e2fe-4517-89cf-650d3329190d.

Wilson-Beattie, Robin. "Learn to #AccessBetter Disability and Sexuality Information with RobinWB!" Robin Wilson-Beattie website. Accessed June 19, 2021. www.robinwb.com/.

Wilson-Beattie, Robin. "My Abortion Story." Disability Visibility Project blog, July 28, 2015. https://disabilityvisibilityproject.com/2015/07/28/guest-blog-post-by-robin-wilson-beattie-my-abortion-story/#:~:text=Robin%3A%20My%20story%20actually%20starts,really%20grueling%20pregnancy%20with%20her.

Yurcaba, Jo. "Law Professor Khiara Bridges Calls Sen. Josh Hawley's Questions about Pregnancy Transphobic." *NBC News*, July 13, 2022. www.nbcnews.com/nbc-out/out-politics-and-policy/law-professor-khiara-bridges-calls-sen-josh-hawleys-questions-pregnanc-rcna38015.

Ziyad, Hari. "My Gender Is Black." *AFROPUNK*, July 12, 2017. https://afropunk.com/2017/07/my-gender-is-black/.

INDEX

abolition medicine, 69–70, 121–122, 136–139
abortion: access, 111; bans, 110–111, 176, 178–182, 184; binary, 21–22; criminalization of, 149, 151, 157, 183; doctor's advice, 131; failed, 160–161; forced, 143, 146; reproductive justice, 26; restrictions on, 58; rights, 16, 29, 118, 148, 156, 177; state surveillance, 94, 156; Wilson-Beattie, 48–49
academy, 12
advocacy: Bill of Rights, 108, 118; bodily autonomy, 89; freedom, 29; genealogies of experience, 13; Isis Tha Savior, 146; limits on people involved, 32; reproductive justice, 50–51; role of storytelling, 3
Afiya Center: abortion care work, 178; community-driven solutions, 109; employs the formerly incarcerated, 128; Jones, 9, 126, 167, 181; work of, 12, 88–89
Afrofuturism, 101
aftermemory, 62, 99
Aiko, Jhené, 71, 73, 148
Alito, Samuel, 148
antiabortion advocates, 86
anti-Black disposability, 39–40
anti-Black society, 135
Arnett, Alvin J., 50
Ashby, Nadine, 46
A Thousand and One, 167–174
Avery, Byllye, 11, 23

Baxter, Mary Enoch Elizabeth (Isis Tha Savior), 28, 125, 146–147
Beloved, 5–6, 10, 30, 75, 84, 129
Benjamin, Ruha, 64
Bey, Marquis, 65
Beyoncé, 175, 176–177
Bhatt, Anand, 163–164, 166
Big Hysto: A Black Womb Revolution, The, 61

235

Birthing Liberation: How Reproductive Justice Can Set Us Free, 162–163
birth justice, 66
Black birthing people: Black maternal mortality, 7; criminalization of, 180; deaths related to abortion, 181–182; drug testing, 159; histories of, 19; incarcerated, 28, 122, 125–126; marginalization of, 35–36, 114; objectified, 142; policing, 28–29, 152–155, 160, 162; reproductive justice, 10–15, 26–27, 76; safety for, 94–95; sterilization of, 112; storytelling, 2
Black children, 102–106, 167, 172
Black disabled birthing people, 48–50, 67–68
Black feminist creativity, 74
Black feminist storytelling, 3–4, 20–21, 25, 32–33, 177, 185
Black futures, 8, 72, 107–108, 149–150
Black life, criminalization of, 170
Black Lives Matter, 150
Black maternal mortality, 7, 31, 34, 52–53, 54–55
Black people: advocacy for, 137; policing, 166; surveillance of, 110–111, 121, 165
Black plus-sized birthing people, 55–57
Black queer birthing people, 42–47
Black queer identity, 25
Black radical imagination, 100–102
Black ratchet imagination, 88–89, 102
Black storytelling, 1–2, 9, 30; changing the narrative, 77; water, 62

Black trans feminism, 65–66
Black Trans Feminism, 65
Black trans people, 40–41
Black Wombholders' Bill of Rights, xxv, 108–110, 117–119
Black women: advocacy for, 89–90; giving birth, 4–5, 6; healing from COVID-19, 92–94; Hill on, 130–131; HIV positive, 51–52; medical experimentation on, 81; naming, 59–60; reproductive justice, 16–18; unmothering, 155–158, 168; violence against, 80
Black Women's Birth Justice, 37, 66
Bland, Sandra, 80
Blige, Mary J., 71, 73
bodily autonomy: advocacy, 89; attacks on, 2, 8, 86; empowering narrative, 90; fight for, 177, 185; forced pregnancy, 110; legislation against gender-affirming care, 65; methodologies for advancing, 13; reproductive justice, 29, 163; restrictions on, 156; sexuality, 87; Shakur, 17; of women and birthing people, 178
botts-ward, reelaviolette, 27, 91–93, 97, 99
Breath, Eyes, Memory, 75
Breedlove, Pauline, 4
Bridges, Khiara, 23, 58–59, 61
Brookins, KB, 44–45
Brooks, Daphne, 88, 176
Browder, Aurelia, 77
Browder, Curtis, 77
Browder, Michelle, 27, 76–80, 82, 84, 88, 99
brown, adrienne maree, 28, 64, 88, 106–107
Brown, Mike, 64, 107
Burrell, Cerita, 7

Bush, Cori, 61
Butler, Octavia, 10, 27, 48, 105–107

Cameron, Daniel, 90
carceral continuum, 147
carcerality, 152
carceral logics, 69, 121–122, 136–137, 139
carceral medicine, 28, 34, 126, 131, 144, 169; birth story, 131, 153; giving birth, 124–126; gynecological care, 144; isolation, 169; subjectivities of Black birthing people, 28; violence of, 34
carceral state, 17, 124, 149–150, 168
carceral system, 130, 145, 171, 173, 187
childbirth: criminalization of, 157; drug testing, 159; dying in, 32, 80; medicalization of, 9, 163; storytellers, 145; waterbreaking, 14; wide range of experience, 162
child protective services (CPS), 154–155, 158, 161–165, 167
Choo, Esther, 13, 24
cisgendered people, 31, 35, 36, 46, 58, 61
Clark-Armstead, Vivian, 53
Clifton, Lucille, 10, 64, 97–98, 107
collective rememory, 63, 74–82
colonial gender system, 37
colonialism, 145
colonial medicine, 41
Colvin, Ciara "Ci Ci," 51
Combahee River Collective, 21
Cooper, Britney, 88–89
Cooper Owens, Deirdre, 20, 23, 81–82
Covid-19: after lockdown, 86, 92; home as sanctuary, 92; incarcerated infection rate, 145; mortality crises, 21; racial health inequities, 2; remote work, 175; rethinking notions of access, 140; systemic racial and gender inequalities, 105
Cox, Kate, 180–181
Crear-Perry, Joia, 24, 66–67
criminalization: abortion, 149, 151, 183; birthing people, 157, 160; Black birth, 173–174; Black birthing people, 155, 162, 180; Black life, 170; Black motherhood, 65, 156; Blackness, 174; Black parents, 165; Black people, 110, 153; of bodies, 69; of pregnancy, 158; of sexually abused, 143
crisis pregnancy centers (CPCs), 111, 112, 179–180
critical fabulation, 19, 20, 62–63
Cross, June, 53
Crossley, Mary, 50

Danticat, Edwidge, 75
DasGupta, Sayantani, 69–70
Davis, Dána-Ain, 10, 23, 94–95, 163
decolonizing reproductive health, 33, 35–39, 42, 62, 66
Dekker, Rebecca, 46
Depo Provera, 65, 112
Dillard, Cynthia B., 63
Dixon Diallo, Dazon, 52
Dobbs, Thomas E., 176
Dobbs v. Jackson: abortion bans, 181, 184; criminalization of birth, 157; Livable Black Futures and, 8; research, 178; *Roe v. Wade* and, 2, 176; Supreme Court, 29, 89, 148

Edinbyrd, Cheryl, 163, 164, 167
Edwards, Frank, 158–159

Eibach, Richard P., 32
endarkened storywork, 63–64, 101
eugenics, 24, 37, 49–51
Evans-Winters, Venus, 18, 19

Falu, Nessette, 24
family separation: anti-Blackness, 174; Black birthing people, 28–29, 125–126; hypersurveillance, 157; policing, 166; prison, 130, 134, 153, 155; remothering, 168; Shakur, 145–146, 185
Fleetwood, Nicole, 147
Floyd, George, 2
formerly incarcerated storytellers, 113, 123–124, 147, 152–153
Fox, Madeline, 9
Freedom Dreams, 101
Freeman, Andrea, 130, 155–156
Friedman, May, 54, 56, 68

Garcia-Hallett, Janet, 25
gender: disrupted during transatlantic slavery, 60; gender identity, 61
gender-affirming care, 65, 86, 104, 115, 178
gendered racial capitalism, 101
gender inequalities, 105
gender non-binary people, 38, 40, 42–45, 73
gender nonconforming, 43
gender progress, 2
gender-queer people, 22, 61, 73
Geronimus, Arline, 153–154
Goodwin, Michele, 156–157
Green, Cheryll, 187
Green, Kai Marshall, 34, 42, 48, 61, 65–66
Guiliani, Rudy, 170
Gumbs, Alexis Pauline, 24

Hahn, Monica U., 137
Haley, Nikki, 53
Hall, DeeDee, 40–42
Hamer, Fannie Lou, 6, 34, 105
Hankinson, Brett, 90
Hansberry, Lorraine, 10
Hargrove, Mystique, 46
Hart, Ericka, 35, 36–37, 66
Hartman, Saidiya, 17, 19, 20, 62–63, 69
Hawley, Josh, 58–59, 61
Hayes, Crystal, 127
healing: botts-ward, 92; Livable Black Futures, 8; medical healing space, 82; remothering, 168; Reproductive Liberation rallies, 86; storytellers, 149; storytelling, 9, 13, 57, 175; storywork, 38
healing justice: Livable Black Futures playlist, 73–76; political strategy, 24; response to trauma, 66
Healing Justice Lineages: Dreaming at the Crossroads of Liberation, Collective Care, and Safety, 66
Herod, Anyika McMillan, 10
Herrera, Lizelle, 180–181
Hersey, Tricia, 175
Hill, DaMaris, 123, 130–131
HIV: Black birthing people, 51–54; living with, 12, 22, 32, 57, 73, 113

Illinois Pro-Choice Alliance, 21
imagination, 64, 100–101, 107
incarcerated birthing people: Black bodies as property, 34; denial of reproductive

autonomy, 28; experiences of, 139–140, 150–151; lack of care for, 122, 133; Shakur, 131; subjectivities of, 125–127
incarcerated mothers, 25
incarcerated patients, 138–139
incarceration: abuse and, 143; dehumanization of, 146; experiences of, 144–145, 149; family separation, 134–135; mass incarceration, 128; reentry into society, 169; Shakur, 16, 121; stigma, 130
inclusivity, 22–23, 73
intersectional invisibility, 32–33, 68, 125
intersectionality: approach, 26; Black futures, 104; medical indignities, 33–34, 54–57, 68; paradigms, 21
In the Wake: On Blackness and Being, 160
Irani, Kayhan, 9
It Gets Messy in Here, 42–43, 61
Iwai, Yoshiko, 69–70

Jackson, Mila, 162, 163–167
Jackson, Rodney, 163–167
Jackson, Temecia, 163–167
James, Joy, 135, 148
Janz, Heidi, 48, 67
Johnson, Kira, 80
Jones, Gayl, 10
Jones, Marsha, 7, 9, 126, 167, 181, 188
Judd, Bettina, 82–83, 97–99

Kaba, Mariame, 64, 117, 119, 125, 136, 157
Kaner, Esther, 137–139
Kelley, Robin D. G., 27, 64, 101, 147

Khan, Zahra H., 69–70
Killing the Black Body, 65, 112
Kincaid, Jamaica, 10
King, Martin Luther, 77
Kouyate, Aminta, 137

Lapeyrolerie, Kortney, 46–47
Leveau, Marie, 123
Lewis-Arnold, Qiana, 7
LGBTQ+ birthing people, 43–44
LGBTQ+ Pride, 176
LGBTQ+ rights, 115
Lind, Emily, 54, 56
Lindsey, Treva, 39–40
Liner Notes for the Revolution, 88
Lithwick, Dahlia, 157
Livable Black Futures: aftermemory, 99; Bill of Rights, 118; Black birthing people, 107–108; bodily autonomy, 7–8; botts-ward, 92; carceral medicine, 122; communal power, 123; formerly incarcerated and, 124, 149; freedom, 102; healing, 8; Mack, 55; medical harm to queer and gender nonbinary, 40; methodology, 22; playlist, 71, 89, 91; reproductive justice, 25, 27–28; storytellers, 14–15, 20, 45, 53; storywork, 9
Lorde, Audre: interdependence, 41–42, 65, 106; on a livable future, 8, 20; on mothering and liberation, 102–104; reproductive justice, 10, 27–28, 102; on self-care, 116; on survival, 142
Louima, Abner, 170
Love, Bettina, 88–89
Lugones, Maria, 37
Lyndon, Audrey, 94–95

Mack, Angela, 55–57, 140–144
marginalization: birthing people, 3, 26, 36, 48, 52, 59–60; identities, 12, 21, 55, 68; mothers of color, 24; political, 154; populations, 126, 163; queer folk, 45; radical *we*, 35; waterbreaking, 15
Martens, China, 24
Martin, Trayvon, 64, 107
Mbembé, Achille, 145
McBride, Renisha, 64, 107
McClain, Dani, 24
McLemore, Monica, 13, 24
medical ableism, 67–68
Medical Apartheid, 81
Medical Bondage, 81
medicine: abolition medicine, 121–122, 136–139; anticolonial approach to, 33; decolonizing, 38–39, 62; disability stigma, 67–68; eugenics in, 24, 50; gynecological, 8, 27, 32, 42; harmful practices, 36; heteronormative, 26, 34, 35, 37, 41; intersectional invisibility, 68; marginalized identities, 12; modern, 14, 81; racialization in, 23; realities of, 182; trans folk, 43; transmisogynoir, 40; weight stigma, 54–56, 61
Megan Thee Stallion, 27, 89, 90, 99
mental health: care transition, 127; concerns around abortion, 183–184; conditions, 36; crisis, 40; disregard for incarcerated, 131; inequity, 122; resources, 115, 147
methodology, 11, 19, 22, 30, 33, 72
Miller, Candi, 183, 184
miscarriage, 5, 47, 95, 146
Morrison, Toni, 4–5, 8, 19, 64, 75

mortality. *See* Black maternal mortality
Mothers of Gynecology, 77, 80, 99
Ms. Foundation for Women, 21
Muganzo-Murphy, Melissa, 61

Nash, Jennifer, 24
National Association to Advance Black Birth, 109
necropolitics, 145
Norplant, 65, 112

oppression: addressing, 59; Black birthing people, 15; Black radical imagination, 100–101; Black women, 21, 106; bodily autonomy, 13; "Break My Soul," 176–177; Butler on dismantling, 106; fight against, 3; gaining control over, 78; gender-nonbinary bodies, 42; healing justice, 24; histories of Black birthing people, 15; holistic, 187; importance of naming, 59; interlocking systems of, 158, 167; organizing against, 176–177; personal power against, 42; possible world out of, 185; racial, 137; refusing, 1; reproductive, 26, 33, 37, 64, 66, 78, 127; reproductive liberation narratives and, 13; resistance, 88, 157; Shakur, 185–187; storywork fighting against, 3; structural, 53; systemic, 24, 171; systems of, 158, 167

Page, Cara, 24, 66, 68–69
Pandit, Eesha, 9
Parable of the Sower, 105–106
patient, 97–98
Perkins-Valdez, Dolen, 10

Perritt, Jamila, 127
Pickens, Theri, 48
Planned Parenthood, 178, 179
playlist, 71–74, 89, 91, 175
Policing the Womb, 156
pregnancy: abortion laws, 176, 182–185; author's daughter, 6; author's experiences, 14; author's loss, 4–5; birthing people, 58; Black birthing people, 109; Black disabled birthing people, 48–50; challenges to receiving abortion care, 179–181; criminalization of Black pregnancy, 155–158; drug testing, 159–160; females resposibility for prevention, 116; forced, 110–111; HIV diagnosis and, 51–54; moral judgement of, 112–113; obesity, 55; people with capacity for, 61; policing, 29, 64; post-partum deaths, 36; queer people, 116; related deaths, 182; reproductive justice, 150; surviving, 32; unwanted, 160–161; while houseless, 154; while incarcerated, 121, 131–133, 145–146, 149, 153, 168–169
Purdie-Vaughns, Valerie, 32
Purdy, Eve, 39

queer birthing people, 42
queer equality, 103
queer folk, 35, 43, 45–46, 115–16; gender-affirming care, 2; medical harm to, 40
queer identity, 25, 27
queer mothers, 24
queerphobia, 35, 51

racial capitalism, 101
racial health inequities, 2
racial inequality, 79, 105
racial inequities, 159
racial injustice, 134
racialization, 23, 42, 54, 107
racial oppression, 137
racial reckonings, 92, 176
racism: Black birthing people, 53; healthcare, 40, 95; institutionalized, 127, 159; medical, 8, 23–24, 32–33, 35–36, 48, 72; oppressive systems, 109; in queer and trans communities, 46; resistance, 187; social stigmas, 41; structural, 172; systemic, 25, 54, 114, 160, 170
radical *we*, 34–35, 38, 48, 65–66
Ralph, Sheryl Lee, 51
ratchetness, 71, 88–89, 90–91
Relf, Mary Alice, 50, 81, 82
Relf, Minnie Lee, 50, 81, 82
reproductive autonomy, 64–65
reproductive justice: abolition medicine, 139; achieving, 24–26; attack on, 2–3; beyond normative frameworks, 39; Black birthing people, 10–15, 26–27, 76; Black feminist storytelling, 3–4, 20–22, 28, 102; bodily autonomy, 29, 163; carcerality and, 28; centering disability in, 50; complexity of, 16; creativity around, 76, 91; full framework of, 131; grammar of, 26–27, 60; history of unfreedom, 29; meaning of, 150; movement, 33–34; narratives, 10, 27; pregnancy, 150; radical movements for, 17; research, 32, 55, 125; resistance, 9, 26; spaces, 90; tenets of, 127, 163, 185; theorizing, 13

reproductive oppression, 64
research: Black identity, 12; Black stories, 31; Cooper Owens, 81; informed by community, 37–38; marginalized populations, 126; qualitative, 25, 63; reproductive justice, 32, 125; storytelling, 9, 153, 155, 162, 177–178; studies, 44; weight stigma, 55
resistance: Afrofuturism, 170; Black lesbians, 24–25; Black storytelling, 2–3, 9, 63, 155; collective, 188; creativity, 73, 85–91; punishment of, 137; rejection of heteronormative logics, 61; reproductive health, 46; reproductive justice, 26; Shakur, 17, 120–123, 185
Rest Is Resistance, 175
Rice, Carla, 54, 56
Roberts, Dorothy, 23, 29, 64–65, 112, 156–157, 165–166, 172
Roberts, Sarah, 159
Rockwell, A. V., 167
Roe v. Wade, 2, 58, 86, 148, 156, 176–177
Rose, Charia, 101
Ross, Loretta, 3, 9, 21, 23, 50–51, 64

Sadiki, Kamau, 16
Sanchez, Sonia, 80
Schaffer, Elijah, 86
Scott, Jill, 140
Scott, Karen, 24, 95, 163
Senate Bill 8, 110–111, 156, 178
sexism, 116
sexual abuse, 143
sexual assault, 113
sexual freedom, 21
sexual health: Black birthing people, 10; Black sexual health, 7, 51, 67–68, 94, 108–109; colonial, heternormative logics, 41; decolonizing, 35, 42; education, 118; generational trauma, 96; harm, 23; inclusion in, 32–33, 37; power of language, 59; queer folk, 45–46; responsibility for pregnancy, 116; waterbreaking, 62; weight stigma, 54
sexuality, 22, 66, 72–73, 87, 89–90, 115
sexual liberation, 27, 74
sexual trauma, 93
Shakur, Assata: *Assata*, 15–18, 28–29, 120–123, 125, 131–135, 185–187; family separation, 145; medical care while incarcerated, 139; medical harm while incarcerated, 142; radical *we*, 34; theory and practice, 101
shame: abortion, 49, 179; body shaming, 72; environment free of, 22, 71, 91, 183; miscarriage, 5; sexual freedom, 87; sexuality, 115; silence, 112–113; social control, 127; weight stigma, 68
Shange, Ntozake, 80
Sharma, Anjana E., 94–95
Sharpe, Christina, 27, 28, 60, 160
Simpson, Monica, 73
Sims, J. Marion, 78, 82
SisterSong, 37, 66, 73
slavery: afterlives of slavery, 154, 171; Black bodies as property, 34; carceral context, 146; critical fabulation, 19; family separation, 165; forced pregnancy, 110;

growing into necropolitics, 145; historical context, 134–135; possesses neoliberal carceral state, 124; state surveillance, 121; transatlantic, 60, 62, 69, 84
Solinger, Rickie, 9, 23, 64
Southern Roots Doula Collective, 37, 66
Spillers, Hortense, 27, 59
Spivak, Gayatri, 19
Stallings, L. H., 88–89
state surveillance, 2, 94, 121, 165
stigma: abortion, 49; Black birthing people, 12; Black disabled birthing people, 50; Black feminist method, 33; disability, 67; environment free of, 22; gynecology, 45; HIV, 51, 53; home births, 162; incarceration, 130; releasing, 72; reproductive health, 10; sexual health, 115; silence, 112–114; social stigmas, 41; weight stigma, 38, 54–57, 61, 68
storytelling. *See* Black storytelling
structural determinants, 66–67
Sufrin, Carolyn, 127
surveillance, 133; of the body, 142; criminalization of poverty and Blackness, 174; discipline, 138; of pregnant people, 156–157, 160; prison, 121; target for, 154, 161; vigilante, 110, 156
Sydnor-Campbell, Tien, 32, 49, 67–68
systemic racism, 25, 54, 114, 160, 170

Tank and the Bangas, 71, 73
Taylor, Breonna, 2, 90
Taylor, Teyana, 167
Thurman, Amber, 181–182, 184
Toliver, S. R., 11–12, 18, 19, 38, 63–64
Tomlinson, Allison, 7
Torn Apart: How the Child Welfare System Destroys Black Families—and How Abolition Can Build a Safer World, 65, 157
Tran, Nhi, 136–137
transatlantic slave trade, 59–60, 62, 69, 84, 146
trans folk, 2, 39–47, 65
transformative justice, 129–130
transphobia, 59, 95, 118
trauma: carceral, 131; family separation, 164; generational, 24, 95, 96; harmfully reframing, 98–99; healing justice, 66; intersectional medical indignities, 57; medical, 4, 96, 142; Morrison on, 75; queer health care, 43; reproductive, 93; reproductive oppression, 26, 33; research team, 127; storytellers, 8, 91; unhealed, 6, 97
Traylor, Masonia, 51

unmothering, 130, 155–159, 164–165, 168

Villarosa, Linda, 24
violence: carceral medicine, 34; obstetric, 8, 10, 33, 72, 163; police, 2, 21, 24, 39, 104; Shakur, 132, 134; socially sanctioned, 80, 125; state, 23, 69; transphobia, 59; vigilante, 110
Voices for Birth Justice, 37, 66

Wade, Sabia, 162–163
Walker, Alice, 97
Washington, Harriet, 20, 81
water, 13–14, 30, 62, 143
waterbreaking: aftermemory and, 99; assaults on family structures, 174; Black feminist creativity, 74; breaking silence, 62, 91; "Break My Soul," 176; childbirth, 14; medical harm, 56; mourning inner child, 93; stories, 15, 30, 144, 153
weight stigma, 38, 54–57, 61, 68
Weinbaum, Alys, 124

Weinberger, Caspar, 50
Wells, Ida B., 105
white supremacy, 26, 33, 88, 104, 157
Wilhemina's War, 53
Williams, Ma'ia, 24
Williams, Serena, 80
Willis, D'Anra, 7
Wilson-Beattie, Robin, 48–49
wombholder, 60–61
Woodland, Ericka, 24, 66

X, Malcolm, 73

Zimba, Helen, 7

Founded in 1893,
UNIVERSITY OF CALIFORNIA PRESS
publishes bold, progressive books and journals
on topics in the arts, humanities, social sciences,
and natural sciences—with a focus on social
justice issues—that inspire thought and action
among readers worldwide.

The UC PRESS FOUNDATION
raises funds to uphold the press's vital role
as an independent, nonprofit publisher, and
receives philanthropic support from a wide
range of individuals and institutions—and from
committed readers like you. To learn more, visit
ucpress.edu/supportus.